Understanding Anesthesia

Understanding Anesthesia

What You Need to Know about
Sedation and Pain Control

Steven L. Orebaugh, M.D.

The Johns Hopkins University Press

Baltimore

The Johns Hopkins University Press
2715 North Charles Street
Baltimore, Maryland 21218-4363
www.press.jhu.edu

Library of Congress Cataloging-in-Publication Data
Orebaugh, Steven L.
Understanding anesthesia : what you need to know
about sedation and pain control / Steven L. Orebaugh.
    p. cm. (A Johns Hopkins Press health book)
Includes bibliographical references and index.
ISBN-13: 978-1-4214-0316-8 (hardback)
ISBN-13: 978-1-4214-0317-5 (pbk.)
ISBN-10: 1-4214-0316-1 (hardcover)
ISBN-10: 1-4214-0317-X (pbk.)
    1. Anesthesia—Popular works. 2. Anesthesiology—Popular works. I. Title.
RD81.074 2011
617.9'6—dc23   2011016275

A catalog record for this book is available from the British Library.

Special discounts are available for bulk purchases of this book.
For more information, please contact Special Sales at 410-516-6936
or specialsales@press.jhu.edu.

The facing page of this book is an extension of this copyright page.

Contents

What are the benefits of regional anesthesia for patients with sleep apnea who undergo surgery?

What is the impact of general anesthesia and opioid pain medications on brain function in the elderly?

Can the use of regional blocks in the elderly lead to an improvement in postoperative complication rates?

How is pain defined?

What are the different types of pain?

How does the nervous system receive and process painful stimuli?

How is pain measured?

How can physicians treat acute pain after surgery?

What are the advantages of a *multimodal* approach to pain management?

Does early treatment of surgical pain reduce the likelihood of chronic pain at the surgery site?

How is an effective pain management service run in a hospital or practice?

What can be done if pain management is inadequate?

Understanding Anesthesia

Chapter 1

Introduction to Anesthesia and Surgery

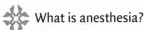 What is anesthesia?

Who is my anesthesiologist?

How will I be prepared for anesthesia?

What are the different techniques of anesthesia?

What is recovery from anesthesia like?

You may be reading this book because you recently had surgery or because you are scheduled for a surgical procedure in the near future. Practically speaking, almost every one of us could benefit from understanding all the events surrounding a surgical procedure, since most people undergo surgery at some point in their lives. In fact, nearly 10 percent of the U.S. population undergoes surgery (or another procedure requiring anesthesia) every year! Anesthesia is a component of most surgical procedures, although it is not always administered by an anesthesiologist or nurse anesthetist. Sometimes, the surgeon provides local anesthesia, with or without a mild degree of sedation.

In this book I primarily discuss anesthesia as it relates to procedures and surgeries that *require* anesthesia and that are to some degree painful. Many books and articles discuss the usefulness and safety of anesthesia. This book is different. I only briefly discuss anesthesia as a profession and touch on issues of safety in the perioperative period (the period immediately before, during, and after surgery). The focus instead is on two forms of anesthesia: general (sleeping) and regional (numbing). I separate these two forms in this book for the purpose of comparing them, but in practice, considering them as separate entities is overly simplistic because the two forms are frequently employed together, in complementary fashion. After considering each technique in isolation, we will see why in practice they are often used together and why this may be beneficial to you for surgery.

Anesthesia can be defined in various ways. For many people, it is synonymous with being unconscious, but anesthesiologists deliver regional anesthesia to thousands of pregnant women in labor every day, most of whom remain awake and are able to participate in the birth process. While many gastrointestinal procedures and other endoscopic interventions require brief anesthesia to ensure comfort during the procedure, the patient feels little or no pain once the procedure has been completed, so the role of regional anesthesia after the procedure is minimal.

Rather than confine the definition of anesthesia to a lack of awareness, let's examine what physicians try to do when they administer anesthesia. In essence, they attempt to make a painful or noxious procedure tolerable, or render a patient unable to perceive the discomfort that accompanies the procedure. The details of your anesthesia will vary with your desires and those of your surgeon, the degree of stimulation during the procedure, the nature of the surgery itself, and even your own physiology and personality.

There are four categories of anesthesia to consider:

1. local anesthesia (the injection of numbing medications only, typically right at the site of the surgical incision)
2. sedation (which, in its extreme, becomes general anesthesia)
3. general anesthesia (complete unresponsiveness, even to pain)
4. regional anesthesia (numbing medications placed in the spine, or in the nerves of the extremities, often used in concert with sedation)

The most basic means of providing an anesthetic might appear to be general anesthesia—putting a patient "to sleep"—but there are other ways of assuring adequate anesthesia. For procedures that are less invasive or painful, mere sedation suffices to keep many patients comfortable. Or, a surgeon or other physician may opt for injecting local anesthetic medications (similar to procaine, or Novocaine) into the area to be incised (cut) or punctured. A "local" is generally used by physicians when sewing up a wound in the emergency department, for example. For many other procedures, sedation is combined with local anesthetic injections to provide pain control and an acceptable lack of awareness of the procedure.

Individual surgeons use different approaches to anesthesia for similar surgical procedures. One surgeon working on a painful foot condition may request intravenous sedation to keep a patient comfortable while he or she numbs the foot with an injection of local anesthesia. A second surgeon may request that the anesthesiologist perform a regional anesthetic block of the entire lower leg, followed by the administration of sedative medications in the operating room. A third surgeon, suspecting that the patient may be unwilling or unable to tolerate a procedure under sedation, might request a general anesthetic for the same procedure. Light degrees of sedation may be provided by an injection or an oral medication given in the preoperative hold area before the procedure begins. When greater degrees of sedation are required, however, anesthesiologists and nurse anesthetists will adjust, or *titrate*, intravenous sedatives into the body throughout the procedure, to more profoundly reduce the level of consciousness.

If you are slated for a relatively superficial operation, then mild sedation, injection of local anesthetic to the affected area, or a combination of the two are most likely to be used for your anesthetic. Such procedures include surgery involving the skin or subcutaneous tissues, minor biopsies, and surgeries on peripheral parts of the body that are easily anesthetized with local anesthetic injections, such as the eyes, fingers, or toes. These types of procedures are quite common, and an important component of modern surgical care is the use of sedation with local anesthesia to provide adequate pain relief and tolerance of minor surgery.

The term *sedation* is rather nonspecific. This process occurs in gradations, as increasing doses of sedative medication are provided (table 1.1). A very light degree of sedation allows you to be awake, or in a drowsy state from which you are easily made alert by someone calling your name or gently touching you. Of importance, you would continue to breathe on your own in this situation, since ventilation is not inhibited.

As sedation deepens, the muscles that maintain an open airway in the neck and the throat may relax and lead to obstruction of airflow. Under these circumstances, an anesthesiologist or nurse anesthetist may need to maintain the airway in an open state, with support of the jaw or chin and assist ventilation if necessary. Appropriate adjustments of sedation are made to avoid greater depths of sedation than required. Patients under this moderate degree of sedation generally respond to physical stimulation, such as gently shaking the shoulder, or loud verbal stimuli, and rarely have any disturbance of blood pressure or cardiac function.

If medication administration continues, "deep" sedation is achieved, and vital systems are significantly affected. Airway obstruction is frequent,

Table 1.1 **Gradations of sedation**

Effects	Wakefulness	Light sedation	Moderate sedation	Deep sedation	General anesthesia
Level of alertness	Alert	Drowsy	Responds to touch	Minimal response	Does not respond
Airway muscles	Intact	Intact	Relaxed	May allow obstruction of airway	Often obstructs
Respiration	Normal	Normal	Slows	May cease	Often ceases
Cardiovascular stability	Stable	Stable	BP may fall	BP often falls	BP falls

Source: Continuum of Depth of Sedation: Definition of General Anesthesia and Levels of Sedation/Analgesia. 2009 Policy Statement by the American Society of Anesthesiologists. Available at www.asahq.org/publicationsAndServices/sgstoc.htm.

Note: BP denotes blood pressure.

breathing efforts become erratic or insufficient, and blood pressure changes are common. This profound degree of sedation requires the presence and attention of an anesthesia provider to ensure your safety and to maintain respiratory and cardiovascular integrity. Today, most hospitals in the United States have sedation protocols that require anesthesia personnel to be in attendance for deep planes of sedation, and health care providers who sedate patients to lesser degrees during invasive procedures are usually required to maintain specific certifications to provide for patient safety.

If the anesthesiologist continues to provide sedative agents to you after you have arrived at this profound degree of somnolence, then general anesthesia is achieved. In this state, loss of consciousness is more profound, and all voluntary responses to stimulation are lost. Respiration and cardiovascular parameters are depressed, and the close monitoring of physiological status is essential. General anesthesia allows much more invasive and painful procedures and surgeries to be performed on your body than can be performed under mere sedation, whether or not local anesthetics are also employed.

Medical students and nurse anesthesia students learn about five factors

Table 1.2 Components of general anesthesia

Alertness	loss of consciousness
Analgesia	prevention of pain
Akinesia	lack of motion
Amnesia	no memory of events
Autonomics	control of vital systems

that compose the state of general anesthesia (table 1.2). These are unconsciousness, failure to perceive pain, relaxed muscles, amnesia of the events of surgery, and close control of vital systems. The drugs used to induce and maintain general anesthesia are administered to provide these five benefits to a patient who is undergoing an invasive or painful procedure. Multiple agents are usually required; the average anesthetic involves the administration of six to ten different pharmacological agents.

On the other end of the anesthesia spectrum, "numbing," or regional, anesthesia procedures can be provided for various operations on extremities and areas such as the breast or the abdominal wall (as in a hernia). Two major classifications of regional anesthesia exist: *neuraxial*, in which local anesthetic medication is placed in the spine to affect the chest wall, abdominal wall, or legs; and *peripheral nerve blockade*, in which the medication is injected near the nerves as they course into the upper or lower extremities. Regional anesthesia is sometimes combined with a general anesthetic, or with sedation, as discussed in chapter 5. Occasionally, patients wish to be wide awake in the operating room, and a regional anesthetic may be conducted with minimal or no sedation to accommodate this request.

Anesthesia is clearly an invaluable tool in the armamentarium of modern health care, allowing invasive and at times miraculous surgeries to be performed while keeping patients comfortable and safe. But who is your anesthesiologist? What type of training has he or she had? Anesthesiology became a board-certified medical specialty in the United States in 1940, with the first fellowships awarded specifically for anesthesia training in 1935. In the very early days of anesthesia, dating to the midnineteenth century, anesthesia was provided by the surgeon. However, the technical requirements of surgery, along with increasing sophistication of anesthesia delivery systems and monitoring, led to the emergence of the specialty that is currently called anesthesiology and perioperative medicine, reflecting the concept that care extends beyond the operating room.

The delivery of anesthesia care in the United States is highly regulated. In most instances, anesthesia is provided to you under the direction of an anesthesiologist, either directly or with a nurse anesthetist. In some cases, a certified nurse anesthetist provides the care in the operating room, under the supervision of the surgeon. In recent years, the nurse anesthesia specialty has lobbied for increasing independence from physician supervision, and in some states their campaign for autonomy has been successful.

The education of an anesthesiologist begins with the standard undergraduate degree, usually a bachelor of science or arts (table 1.3). He or she may elect to perform graduate work to achieve a master's degree, but most people who plan to become anesthesiologists proceed directly to the four-year medical school program, earning an M.D. or D.O. degree. The next step is internship, which may be an integral part of the anesthesiology residency, or may be performed independently, in an entirely different hospital system. Increasingly, the integral internship, with a specific curriculum designed to enhance subsequent anesthesia learning, is being favored. In either case, the internship is multidisciplinary, with required rotations in surgery, internal medicine, and acute care, such as emergency medicine and critical care medicine. This is often rounded out with experience in obstetrics and gynecology, ambulatory medicine, and anesthesia itself.

After the intern year has been completed, the three-year residency program begins. The educational component is dictated by the Residency Review Committee of the Accreditation Council of Graduate Medical Education, and requires certain amounts of time (and case experience) in various subspecialties of anesthesiology, such as obstetrics, cardiac and thoracic surgery, and regional anesthesia, along with related areas in which anesthesiologists should have expertise, such as the post-anesthesia care unit (PACU, or recovery room), acute pain therapy, chronic pain management, and critical care medicine. Electives are permitted in the third year, to allow a degree of specialization as the resident prepares to go into private or academic practice. In certain areas, extra training in a fellowship is required to obtain subspecialty certification. Currently, these subspecialties include critical care medicine, chronic pain management, and cardiac anesthesia. Other areas in which a fellowship is useful, both to obtain the necessary experience and competence and to enhance the anesthesiologist's

Table 1.3 Typical pathway for education and certification of an anesthesiologist in the United States

1. Undergraduate degree (4 years)

2. Medical school attendance (4 years): M.D. or D.O. degree

3. Internship (1 year): independent or associated with a residency program

4. Residency in anesthesiology (lasting 3 years after internship)

5. Optional fellowship for subspecialty training (1 to 3 years, depending on subspecialty): examples include cardiac, obstetric, pediatric, and regional anesthesia as well as critical care medicine and chronic pain medicine

6. Written board examination

7. Oral board examination

8. Optional subspecialty (fellowship) examination

9. Maintenance of certification process

ability to obtain a position in the field, include obstetric anesthesia, pediatric anesthesia, and regional anesthesia. (Some or all of these areas may become board-certified subspecialties in the future.) Research fellowships are a popular option for academic physicians.

After successful completion of training in anesthesiology, the physician-anesthesiologist is required to undergo written examination. After successfully completing the written test, the candidate must also take and pass an oral examination. Those who elect to take a fellowship in one of the formal subspecialties must also take a subspecialty examination in that field. Although older anesthesiologists were initially "certified for life," graduates after the year 2000 are required to recertify every ten years. In addition, those certified must participate in ongoing programs of continuing education and documentation of experience to remain certified.

Once education has been formally completed, anesthesiologists choose between working in the private sector or remaining in academic medicine. In academic medicine, in addition to practicing anesthesiology, the anesthesiologist would perform research and publish medical articles as well as teach medical students and residents. The large majority of physicians in most specialties enter private practice, since academic slots are limited, and most physicians chose medicine as a profession to provide patient care, not to teach or do research.

You may wonder who your anesthesiologist actually works for. At a university hospital, the physicians are usually in an academic practice, and they may have a faculty appointment, such as assistant professor, or professor, of anesthesiology. Thus, they are employed by the university hospital system itself, or by a physician practice plan that includes the physicians at that teaching hospital. At private hospitals, and in freestanding surgical centers, the anesthesiologists usually are members of a group that has contracted with the hospital or institution to provide the anesthesia service for their surgical patients. Sometimes, large contract management entities control the contracts, employing anesthesiologists and nurse anesthetists, whereas in other situations, physician groups have obtained the contracts. In a few instances, an individual anesthesiologist (or nurse anesthetist) will be employed by a surgeon, or by a facility owned by one or a group of surgeons. In some parts of the country, anesthesiologists working in the same hospital may be individual practitioners, competing to work with different surgeons.

Although physician education in anesthesia is relatively uniform, the means by which patient information is conferred to anesthesiologists to prepare for anesthesia, and to make certain that patients have been screened for unsafe conditions, is not. Some larger groups and hospitals conduct a *preoperative clinic* in which patients slated for surgery are seen days or even weeks ahead of time, to allow ample time to optimize care for medical conditions or to perform diagnostic studies, if needed. For many smaller groups this approach is not an option, and the preoperative visit may be conducted in the operating room area during the anesthesiologist's workday, on an as-needed basis. Because most surgeries are performed on an ambulatory, or outpatient, basis today, access to the patient has become more limited than in decades past, when patients were hospitalized before surgery, permitting a preoperative evaluation on the floor the day before surgery.

Many groups, particularly those who see a preponderance of ambulatory surgery patients, gather preoperative information by phone screening or use of the Internet. In the latter case, patients fill out the medical history on an electronic form, which can be accessed by the anesthesiologist.

If there are questions or concerns, a visit can be arranged, or surgery is delayed until the relevant medical conditions have been addressed. Preoperative clinics and preoperative screening have been shown to reduce last-second surgery postponements and cancellations, thus improving both efficiency of operating room utilization and patient satisfaction.

It is very important for you to discuss underlying medical conditions with your anesthesiologist, since such conditions, even if well controlled, may affect the amount and type of anesthesia provided. This information will help the provider make appropriate adjustments, and let him or her know what additional risks anesthesia may pose for you. In general, if you have a condition that requires ongoing medical treatment, you should mention it. Any medical problem involving the heart or lungs should be included, as well as neurological conditions. Likewise, endocrine, metabolic, blood, and gastrointestinal diseases should be noted. If you have had anesthesia before, you should discuss any adverse reactions or unpleasant symptoms that resulted, such as an allergic response or postoperative nausea. This information allows the physician to make alterations in the anesthetic plan to keep you safe and make you more comfortable.

Thus, your anesthesiologist will learn about you and your medical history. He or she will then spend additional time at your bedside immediately before surgery, confirming the information in the chart, expanding on it, and asking additional questions specific to your medical and surgical conditions, medications, allergies, and responses to prior anesthetics. In addition, the anesthesiologist will carry out a brief physical examination. After these steps have been taken, an intravenous catheter is inserted, and consent is obtained for the anesthesia to be conducted. I will focus more on this period in the perioperative process when I discuss the administration of general anesthesia.

An explanation of the anesthetic choices will be offered during the process of obtaining consent. In some cases, there is no real choice. For instance, when your tonsils are removed, or your gallbladder is removed with a laparoscopic procedure, there is little choice but to use general anesthesia. If you have a normal pregnancy and go into labor, and you desire pain relief, regional anesthesia in the form of an epidural will be offered, since general anesthesia might depress the fetus. However, many operations may be conducted under either regional anesthesia or general anesthesia, or a combination of the two.

It would be inappropriate to suggest that patients be presented a "menu" of potential anesthetic types on the day of surgery from which they can order whatever they choose. The anesthesiologist must consider the type of surgery, the desires of the surgeon, and the safety of the patient in arriving at an anesthetic plan. He or she will then present this plan to the patient. The details will also depend to some extent on the provider's experience and comfort level with various types of anesthetics. What is safest and most effective in one doctor's hands may not be so in the hands of a different anesthesiologist. Sometimes different choice of technique is possible, and sometimes it is not. For any painful surgery, however, it is reasonable to ask how the anesthesiologist will manage postoperative pain, and if a regional nerve block is applicable for this purpose.

Trying to decide which type of anesthesia you should have, when choices are possible, may be difficult. Many patients turn to a spouse or other loved one for advice. Others prefer "whatever the surgeon wants" (surgeons often have no preference, and they leave this decision to the patient and the anesthesiologist). A great many patients simply state: "Just put me out, doc," or "I don't want to know anything. Put me to sleep." These kinds of statements suggest that the patient was not well prepared to face the question of anesthesia choice, or would prefer not to deal with it during this stressful period. This book was written to provide you with information that will make it easier to know in advance which type of anesthesia you would prefer, if a choice is indeed possible. To make an informed decision, you must understand, for example, the benefits of regional anesthesia as a sole intervention, or, more commonly, in concert with unconsciousness in the operating room. As we shall see, regional anesthesia offers various benefits, both psychological and physiological, that can be integrated into the anesthesia plan while still allowing for the common preference to be unaware of events in the operating room.

You should not show up for surgery without giving some thought to anesthesia. If you ask just a few questions of the surgeon or the surgical staff, you will likely get useful information about the choices of anesthesia available for your particular procedure. The anesthesiologist can clarify these choices for you. In my experience, many patients are reluctant to ask for alternatives when it comes to the anesthetic plan. However, the tendency in anesthesia, as in all of medicine, is to be more forthcoming with explanations and alternatives than was the case a few decades ago, in a more paternalistic era.

When you sign permission for anesthesia, you are attesting that you have been provided information that allows you to understand the procedure, its risks and benefits, and the alternatives. If you don't believe that you have been given enough information to make this judgment, don't sign. Ask for more input. Most providers are happy to explain which anesthetic options exist in your situation, and why they may favor one technique over another in light of certain underlying medical conditions or your previous reactions to anesthesia. Sometimes, the anesthesiologist may not be well trained in or comfortable with a certain technique that you request or have heard about and will have to tell you frankly that a different technique is safest and most reliable in his or her hands.

We have now considered the methods of providing anesthesia, including general, regional, sedation, local, or some combination of these, for the surgical procedure. But after surgery has been concluded and you are wheeled to the recovery room, how is the recovery from anesthesia optimized? This process actually starts in the operating room. The anesthesia provider will gauge your need for systemic pain medications by your body weight and by your vital signs during the surgery and will provide these medications throughout the procedure, with an increasing emphasis on the pain relief aspects of the anesthetic as the procedure winds down. Some indicators, such as high blood pressure, increased heart rate, and rapid respiratory rate, show that the body is sensing pain and is responding to the surgical stimulus.

Even when a patient is in a deep state of unconsciousness, anesthesiologists expect a degree of surgical "stimulation." Indeed, without the physiological adaptation of increased blood pressure in response to the surgical stimulus, anesthesia would frequently result in a dangerously low blood pressure. As your anesthesia is lightened, your sympathetic (fight or flight) nervous system begins to show signs that stress is being perceived, such as increases in heart rate, blood pressure, and respiratory rate. The opioid components of anesthesia (morphine, fentanyl, or hydromorphone) are of particular importance at this time, to control that response of your nervous system and to allow you to awaken with minimal discomfort.

As you regain consciousness, a sense of confusion and disorientation is common. The anesthesiologist or anesthetist will repeatedly orient you and let you know that you are safe and that surgery has been completed. By the time you arrive in the recovery room, you will usually be able to perceive what's happening around you. Pain that you did not sense when you woke up in the OR may make itself known to you in the PACU (post-anesthesia care unit or recovery room). The nurse at the bedside will "take report" about you and your surgical case from the anesthesia provider, and ask you about pain and other unpleasant feelings, such as cold or nausea, that you may be experiencing. The anesthesiologist will order medications for pain and nausea, as well as address other issues such as shivering and high or low blood pressure.

Nurses who take over your care in the recovery room, under the guidance of the anesthesiologist, are specially trained in post-anesthesia nursing. They are committed to providing the best possible care during the recovery period. Like anesthesia providers, they work under the guidelines established by specialty societies, and they pursue continuing education along these lines. Post-anesthesia nursing is considered a critical care nursing specialty, like intensive care nursing, and requires a higher degree of training than for basic medical-surgical nursing.

The ratio of nurses to patients in the PACU is higher than it is in the hospital ward, or in the ambulatory surgical unit. Certain criteria must be met before surgical patients are transferred from the PACU to the next phase of recovery. These criteria relate to wakefulness, blood pressure, oxygen levels in the bloodstream, breathing, and strength. A patient is not transferred to the ambulatory surgical unit, also called phase 2 recovery, until he or she has met the requirements described in table 1.4. The same criteria govern whether an inpatient who has undergone surgery may be transferred to the hospital ward or unit in which he or she will continue to convalesce.

The process of "waking up" may take a few minutes or even several hours, depending on your physiology and susceptibility to anesthesia as well as on the amount of opioid medication required for pain control. Repeated doses of pain medication in the recovery room can be viewed as a "second anesthetic" because they cause patients to become drowsy and nauseated, and often to completely forget events that occur there. Most surgeons avoid speaking to patients in the recovery room, because they are well aware that the patient will not remember the conversation; instead, they speak to loved ones in the surgical waiting room. As we will see, avoiding this "second anesthetic" is among the most favorable aspects of regional anesthesia, since patients generally awaken with minimal or no pain and therefore no need for opioid medications.

Although the recovery room stay is necessary for many surgical patients, it may be possible to skip this stop under certain circumstances. Most people would be much happier awakening at the end of surgery without pain or nausea, being able to immediately think clearly and talk, and bypass

Table 1.4 **Main components of post-anesthesia care unit (PACU)
or recovery room discharge criteria**

1. **Wakefulness.** Is the patient awake enough to respond?

2. **Blood pressure stability.** Is the blood pressure close to the baseline, or starting blood pressure, recorded before surgery and anesthesia began?

3. **Oxygen saturation.** Is the oxygen level in the bloodstream close to the patient's baseline?

4. **Respiratory effort.** Is the patient awake enough to provide strong breathing effort?

5. **Muscle strength.** Have the muscles sufficiently recovered strength to allow the patient to breathe and function?

the PACU to go straight back to the ambulatory surgical unit, where their loved ones are waiting to see them. This is the goal of ambulatory surgical programs, and it is achievable in many cases. For brief surgeries, in which pain has been well managed, achieving the landmarks necessary to bypass the PACU is not difficult.

Over the last decade or so, the process of *PACU bypass* has been found safe and reliable as long as the patient meets a number of physiological criteria—in fact, the same criteria he or she must meet at the end of a PACU stay. How is this accomplished? Anesthesiologists are able to employ fast-acting, rapid-recovery agents and emphasize nausea control and pain management. Newer anesthetics, both the gaseous and the intravenous varieties, allow more rapid emergence from deep states of unconsciousness and a much shorter period of "anesthetic hangover." In addition, significant progress has been made in controlling those effects of anesthesia and surgery that make going home the day of the procedure difficult.

The most common reasons for prolonged stays after ambulatory procedures are pain and nausea. Control of these two problems has become an important emphasis in ambulatory anesthesia, and much research has been devoted to them. Drugs that reduce nausea fit into seven different categories. In many ambulatory surgical settings, specific drugs that act by different pathways are employed together as prophylaxis to reduce the risk of postoperative nausea, rather than waiting for it to occur and then attempting to treat it in the postoperative period. You should tell the anesthesiologist, in the preoperative interview, whether nausea has been problematic for you after prior surgeries, so he or she can focus on providing you with prophylactic medications to prevent nausea.

Pain control is an essential feature of all anesthetics, whether ambulatory or not. Certainly, the anesthesiologist prefers to control your pain from the outset if you are slated to return home the same day; for the inpatient, the anesthesiologist has more time to titrate pain medications to the level of discomfort during the recovery room stay and on the inpatient unit. Just as several pathways can be exploited for prevention or treatment of nausea, pain can be controlled through multiple modes. These include regional anesthesia nerve blocks and various types of medications. Employing different modalities is called *multimodal analgesia*, a concept that has been a central tenet of acute pain management in recent years. It means using several different modalities of therapy simultaneously to control pain, including intravenous and oral medications as well as regional anesthetic blocks. Nerve blocks are discussed in detail in chapters 5–7, and their overall place in pain management are explored further in chapter 10.

This brief introduction to anesthesia has covered the components of anesthesia, described who your anesthesiologist is and how he or she will learn about you, and considered what aspects of your perioperative care fall under his or her control. After a brief discussion of the history of anesthesia in the next chapter, chapter 3 moves on to the topic of general anesthesia and its consequences in some detail, followed by discussion of the two major types of regional anesthesia. After reviewing the specific regional anesthesia needs of some defined subsets of patients, chapter 10 explores how general and regional anesthesia are frequently integrated to provide optimal postoperative outcomes for patients, in concert with other pain management techniques in the multimodal approach.

Chapter 2

A Brief History of Anesthesia

 How long has anesthesia been available?

What was surgery like before anesthesia?

How did the discovery of anesthesia influence surgery?

Who is credited with the first uses of surgical anesthesia?

How did general anesthesia and regional anesthesia come into common use at the same time?

What would life be like without anesthesia? One need not delve far into the past to arrive at a time when there was no anesthesia to make surgery tolerable. In fact, though surgical procedures were performed for thousands of years, it was not until the 1840s that techniques were developed to anesthetize patients, keeping them unconscious and unable to feel pain during surgery.

General anesthesia was a Holy Grail, for practitioners of surgery and patients alike, until the mid-nineteenth century. Those who underwent surgery, either because of disease processes or because of injury, were subject to unimaginable pain and suffering. Descriptions of these patients' experiences can be very disturbing because of the vivid pictures of suffering they portray. Many patients with diseases avoided surgery until it was no longer possible to ignore an expanding abscess, tumor, or malformation. Some patients preferred death to the horrible pain of surgery without anesthesia. Stark reminders of the fear and agony associated with the surgical process are the hooks, ropes, and fasteners evident in historical surgical theaters, where operations were often conducted in front of an audience. Strong ties and muscular attendants were needed to hold patients in place during operations, so frantic were these traumatized patients from the pain caused by scalpels, saws, and probes. Some surgeons lamented the terrible pain they caused while others found patients' protests to be a nuisance and denied the significance of pain in the surgical process. In actuality, surgical therapy was severely limited by the pain it caused, and, for many patients, the "cure" was to be feared more than the disease itself.

It is no wonder, then, that healers searched for thousands of years for ways to alleviate pain in general, and specifically the pain inherent in surgical treatment. Many remedies were used over the centuries to make operative pain tolerable. These included mandragora (from the mandrake plant), mixtures of herbs and poppies (which contain opium), hypnosis, ethyl alcohol, and even rubbing the area to be operated on with ice. None of these means of anesthetizing was particularly effective in the surgical realm, and the search continued for a means to control pain during invasive procedures.

By the mid-nineteenth century, the gaseous chemicals that eventually emerged as general anesthetics were already well known to scientists and laypeople alike. In fact, even their properties of reversibly rendering animals or people unconscious, or at least insensible to pain, were understood. Paracelsus, the famed physician of the sixteenth century who is credited with ushering in the era of modern medicine, had described ether in that period as "sweet oil of vitriol." Humphry Davy, an eminent chemist of the late eighteenth and early nineteenth century, popularized nitrous oxide, a compound that had been discovered in 1773. He noted that this colorless, odorless gas could briefly relieve pain and even suggested its possible use for surgery in a textbook he wrote on the subject. He deemed it "laughing gas."

But these ideas lay fallow in the developing profession of medicine until the 1840s, when four American doctors—two dentists, one academician, and one rural general practitioner—began to apply these important compounds to the relief of pain during operations. Each man helped lay the foundation of the new field of anesthesiology that would develop in the wake of their insightful efforts. Unfortunately, bitter rivalries developed among these men in their attempts to claim credit for this remarkable discovery, and controversy reigned in the years following the first publicized applications of general anesthetics.

Crawford Long, a general practitioner in rural Georgia, appears to have been the first physician to employ diethyl ether, commonly called ether, to reduce the pain of both surgery and childbirth. This beloved country doctor began administering ether as an inhalant in 1842 during a minor surgical procedure on the neck of a friend. He later also applied it successfully to reduce the pain of childbirth. Long continued to use ether in his practice intermittently thereafter. Unfortunately, he did not keep accurate records of his remarkable deed, nor did he attempt to report this incredible feat to the medical community of his day. In fact, he did not publicize it in any way and for this reason is seldom given credit for the discovery of anesthesia. In later years, when the controversy over the advent of anesthesia was raging, Long began to describe his early experiences, and his name became associated with the introduction of the new medical process. He was certainly a leader in the field, who practiced a humanistic style of medicine in advance of his contemporaries.

Soon thereafter, a Connecticut dentist named Horace Wells began to apply nitrous oxide to patients in his Hartford practice to ameliorate the pain of dental procedures. He had become aware of nitrous oxide from its unseemly reputation, which it had acquired when its abuse potential became obvious in the early nineteenth century. On city streets, itinerant hucksters would sell brief inhalations of nitrous oxide to provide a thrill. Traveling shows moved from town to town, sensationalizing the inebriation that occurred when volunteers from the audience inhaled this gas. A humorous spectacle ensued as they jumped and cavorted across the stage in front of a bemused crowd. So insensible were these volunteers, for a few minutes, that injury did not seem to cause pain. At just such a show, this phenomenon was noted by Horace Wells as blood dripped from the injured knee of an acquaintance. The dentist arranged for removal of his own decayed tooth under the influence of inhaled nitrous oxide and declared that he sensed no pain. He then eagerly began to apply the gas in his dental practice.

Wells found that nitrous oxide worked very well to control the pain of tooth extractions in his patients. He popularized the idea of "painless dentistry" in Hartford, and his reputation began to grow. Another young dentist, William Morton, came to Hartford to learn Wells' techniques, and the two were briefly in partnership. Morton's chief interest at the time was in sharing a business venture with Wells, which involved a new compound for filling and rebuilding teeth. The partnership did not last, but Wells remained determined to demonstrate the potential of nitrous oxide for relieving surgical pain.

He was granted his opportunity in January 1845, at the prestigious Massachusetts General Hospital. On an afternoon set aside for the operation, a tooth extraction, Wells presented his case before a skeptical audience of physicians, academics, and other interested parties convened by one of the founding fathers of the hospital, a surgeon named John Collin Warren. The hopeful dentist carefully applied the gas as the onlookers watched curiously, and the patient appeared to lapse into unconsciousness. Tension built in the room as he reached into the patient's mouth and grasped an offending tooth. But just as he removed the tooth, the patient cried out in pain. Not surprisingly, Wells was jeered by the audience. The demonstration had been an abject failure, and Wells never recovered from his humiliation. The patient himself, however, later reported that he had experienced no pain, and therefore nitrous oxide had probably played the role intended. Nevertheless, the learned audience was quick to dismiss Wells and his anesthetic gas. Some years later, Horace Wells became an addict to the nitrous oxide that he had helped to introduce to the world. He was arrested for a bizarre incident in which he assaulted a woman on the streets of New York City, spattering acid on her. After his conviction, he was jailed and fell into deep despair. In his cell, he reportedly slit his wrist and took his own life.

William Morton, the other New England dentist who played a vital role in the birth of anesthesia, became interested in the anesthetizing properties of ether, a vapor much more potent than nitrous oxide. This substance was capable of providing a more profound degree of unconsciousness, allowing complete insensibility during painful procedures. Because of its high degree of potency, a mixture of ether with air was commonly applied to the patient or animal to be anesthetized, ensuring continued administration of oxygen. Nitrous oxide, on the other hand, to be effective as an anesthetic, had to be administered in high concentrations, excluding other gases, and only for short periods before the body became starved for oxygen. The admixture of ether with air could be insufflated for much longer periods, and with a fair degree of safety.

Morton acquired experience with ether as an anesthetic agent, first in animals and later in his dental practice. He became convinced that it could be widely applied to control surgical pain. He, too, arranged a public demonstration, in front of a similarly skeptical crowd at the Massachusetts General Hospital, about a year after the debacle staged by Horace Wells. The surgical procedure was to be the removal of a neck tumor, which was carried out in an amphitheater that became known thereafter as "The Ether Dome." Morton arrived late for the scheduled procedure, earning the ire of the attending surgeon, once again Dr. Warren. However, Morton was able to successfully anesthetize the patient, making use of a newly devised ether inhalation flask. After resection of the tumor without a movement or protest from the patient, Warren proclaimed to the astonished audience, "Gentlemen, this is no humbug." Such was the introduction of general anesthesia to an anxious, waiting world.

A fourth important character in the complex drama surrounding the advent of anesthesia in the 1840s was the geologist, metallurgist, and Harvard physician Charles Jackson. Jackson was well known in Boston and throughout the nation for his multiple talents, and he provided Morton useful advice on the chemical nature of ether and its safe administration. This advice allowed Morton to successfully use the vapor as an anesthetic. Jackson initially distanced himself from William Morton. He found the dentist's overt attempts to profit from the advent of surgical anesthesia to be morally reprehensible. Camouflaging ether with scented additives, Morton attempted to obtain a patent for the readily available chemical so he could reap a fortune for this astounding advance in medicine.

Later Jackson would work hard to claim some if not all of the credit for the initial use of ether in an operation, asserting that Morton was simply doing his bidding. The famed academician spent much of the rest of his life trying to convince medical societies in the United States and abroad that he was responsible for the initial administration of ether to provide anesthesia for surgery. After years of attempting to manipulate public opinion regarding the relative contributions of the two dentists and himself, Charles Jackson suffered a severe stroke and spent the last years of his life unable to communicate.

Thus, the initial use of these two most humane substances for the relief of surgical pain was marked by controversy, avarice, and heartbreak. This remarkable advance in medicine was not readily attributable to one single individual. Long, Wells, Morton, and Jackson are all remembered for their contributions. Their efforts culminated in the foundation of a new medical specialty. As anesthesia advanced in complexity and sophistication, many surgeries could be performed that had been impossible before anesthesia. Thereafter, the two specialties of surgery and anesthesiology would grow in tandem, each driving the other forward into new arenas.

Soon after the first public display of ether as surgical anesthesia in the United States, James Simpson of Scotland discovered the pleasant anesthetizing effects of chloroform, which he used to control the pain of labor and childbirth. Initial controversy surrounding its use in this setting subsided substantially when Queen Victoria of England asked for it to control the pain of her labor. Innumerable advances attended the use of anesthetics in the second half of the nineteenth century, including the development of sophisticated insufflation devices to control inhaled anesthetic concentrations, devices to enhance the safety of patients, and the first textbook of anesthesia.

During the twentieth century, the specialty of anesthesiology became an indispensable component of modern medical practice. Placing tubes into the trachea for delivery of anesthetic gases and control of ventilation became routine, anesthetic machines were developed to apply precise mixtures of gases, and monitors for ensuring patient safety increased in number and sophistication. New drugs were developed to provide instantaneous loss of consciousness when delivered intravenously, and the halogenated hydrocarbons (such as halothane) were synthesized and found to be effective inhaled anesthetics, safer and less flammable than earlier gases, which they supplanted. Societies were founded to guide the development of anesthesia and perpetuate the specialty's emphasis on patient protection. At the beginning of the twenty-first century, when the United States Institute of Medicine declared that one hundred thousand patients per year were dying needlessly from medical errors, anesthesiology was mentioned prominently as an exemplary specialty, receiving accolades from the institute for its emphasis on patient safety, its commitment to vigilance, and the prevention of medical errors.

Anesthesia need not involve the loss of consciousness, or even sedation. Anesthesiologists frequently rely on regional anesthesia techniques to provide insensibility to the pain inflicted by surgical trauma. Like general anesthesia, regional anesthesia is a product of the nineteenth century. All regional anesthetics involve the injection of drugs that temporarily inactivate nerves at the site of injection. By binding to certain ion channels on nerve fibers, these drugs, the local anesthetics, stop electrical impulses from traveling down the nerves, thus interrupting sensibility and muscle control. This results in a temporary loss of sensation as well as muscle weakness. The first such drug to be used was cocaine, when Karl Koller, a Viennese intern, employed the drug topically to numb the cornea for eye surgeries in 1884.

When physicians recognized that cocaine could produce a loss of sensation if applied to the membranes of the eyes, nose, or mouth, its potential for use in surgery became obvious. Cocaine was applied to the nerves of the upper extremity under direct vision through a surgical incision by William Halsted in 1884. Although this methodology was impractical, it showed that local anesthetics could provide a new type of anesthesia, one that did not require a loss of consciousness. The next step involved the injection of local anesthetic solutions through the skin, first described by Georg Hirschel and Diedrich Kulenkampff in 1911. A dozen years prior to this, in 1899, August Bier, in Germany, had described the application of cocaine to the spinal nerves, producing a short-lived "spinal" anesthetic. Over half a century later, Martinez Curbelo of Cuba reported using a catheter in the spine to provide a continuous form of "epidural" anesthesia, allowing pain control for long periods. Descriptions of other types of nerve blocks appeared throughout the twentieth century. Even as late as the 1990s, new techniques were being described, and subtle variations of block techniques continue to be cataloged to this day.

A spectrum of local anesthetic medications was developed, with a range of durations from less than an hour to half a day or more, depending on the site of application, the concentration, and the dose of the agent. Having these options has allowed great flexibility in selecting anesthesia for various surgeries and for postoperative pain relief. Some of these drugs perform more effectively for spinal blockade, some for epidural blocks, and some for peripheral nerve blockade. A few local anesthetic drugs, such as lidocaine, can be used in all these scenarios. Additives such as epinephrine (adrenaline) can be employed to prolong the effect of certain local anesthetic drugs. The use of catheters in concert with epidural blockade and with peripheral nerve blockade was successfully applied in the mid-twentieth century to allow even more prolonged pain relief, lasting several days after surgery was completed.

Thus, general anesthesia and regional anesthesia developed in parallel. Although some anesthesiologists adhere tightly to one or the other technique in certain situations, most are skilled in both. General anesthesia and regional anesthesia are frequently used together, with the regional anesthesia affording patients a more comfortable emergence from general anesthesia, a reduction in the doses of medications used to provide the general anesthetic, and minimizing certain undesirable side effects. Some form of regional anesthesia is used in nearly one-third of all surgeries in this country and may be offered to you for many different types of surgical procedures. As we shall see, general anesthesia is indispensable for certain types of surgery, and it could not be supplanted by regional techniques.

For other procedures, a choice of either regional or general anesthesia is possible. In light of the anesthesiologist's skills and training, the nature of the procedure, and your desires as a patient, he or she will discuss these possibilities with you in the preoperative period. Either type of anesthesia can provide maximal comfort with no awareness of what takes place in the operating room. How the two techniques differ; their advantages, disadvantages, and side effects; and how they may be used in a complementary fashion will become clear in later chapters.

Chapter 3
General Anesthesia

 What does general anesthesia entail?

How is general anesthesia different from sedation?

What can I expect before surgery with general anesthesia?

Why do I need an IV (intravenous cannula) for an anesthetic?

What is the purpose of all those monitors?

What happens to patients' breathing under general anesthesia?

How will my anesthesiologist keep me safe under anesthesia?

What are the most common side effects of general anesthesia?

Almost three-quarters of surgeries performed in the United States today occur on an outpatient basis. Ambulatory surgical patients usually meet their anesthesiologist only a few minutes before the planned surgical procedure is to begin. While the anesthesiologist usually has information about the patient's medical history from a preoperative screening taken over the phone or by computer, or from a preoperative evaluation clinic, the patient and the anesthesiologist seldom have the opportunity to meet each other before the day of surgery. This unfortunate situation is relatively new, and although certainly cost effective, it does little for the doctor-patient relationship.

A decade or so ago, most patients stayed in the hospital at least overnight before surgery. The anesthesiologist would visit the patient on the afternoon before the procedure to discuss concerns, answer questions, and provide reassurance. He or she would also arrange for specific preoperative therapy, which used to include injecting a relatively potent mixture of sedative medications to provide sedation before the patient even left the hospital room for the journey to the operating room. Today, the anesthesiologist must do all these things in a few short minutes before the operation. For the anesthesiologist, it is difficult, if not impossible, to develop a trusting, caring relationship with a patient in just five or ten minutes of conversation before surgery. On the other hand, when the patient has the benefit of an inpatient preoperative visit and is able to greet the anesthesiologist again the next day, as the operation is about to begin, he or she will likely see the anesthesiologist as an ally. If the patient meets the anesthesiologist only once, for a brief conversation, then this physician may be no more memorable than the six or eight other people the patient meets in the operating room that day.

Since the ambulatory (outpatient) model of efficient surgical care has made the formal preoperative visit in your hospital room somewhat unusual, you can expect a relatively intense period of examination and discussion when you meet the anesthesiologist on the day of surgery (table 3.1). The anesthesiologist will ask questions related to your respiratory, cardiac, gastrointestinal, blood, and metabolic systems. Medications and allergies are noted, and questions about recent food or fluid intake will be asked. Appropriate preoperative medications will be administered, and other medications are prepared for administration during surgery (table 3.2). A brief physical examination follows, in which the anesthesiologist pays attention to dental structures, throat and neck characteristics, and lung and heart sounds. While many questions asked may seem redundant, medical professionals are taught to be thorough *and* repetitive. If someone has inadvertently recorded a drug allergy inappropriately, or written illegibly, it could have dire consequences for a patient as care proceeds.

After the history and physical examination comes a discussion about the anesthetic. This discussion will include any potential options (such as whether a nerve block would be useful or advisable), risks and benefits of the anesthetic to be utilized, and what you can expect in the perioperative process. While doctors have no wish to intimidate patients regarding the risks of anesthesia, the trend is to be frank at the bedside about what can go wrong. This trend reflects the emphasis in medicine on truly "informed" consent. Surgical patients need to understand exactly what it is that they

Table 3.1 How the anesthesiologist evaluates the patient before surgery

Confirms the patient's identity and the proposed procedure.

Obtains medical history and performs brief physical examination.

Reviews laboratory results (if necessary, given patient's history, age, proposed surgery).

Explains and discusses anesthesia and any options available (spinal or general anesthesia, nerve blocks, and any other special modalities).

Obtains consent for the proposed anesthetic.

Marks the body part to be involved in procedures (specifically for a nerve block; otherwise, the surgeon usually provides these marks).

Table 3.2 A sampling of medications often used in the period before surgery

Purpose	Examples
Treat pre-existing medical conditions	antihypertensives (for blood pressure)
	anti-anginal agents (for coronary disease)
	bronchodilator inhalers (for asthma)
Prevent nausea	ondansetron (Zofran)
	scopolamine patch
Prevent pain and inflammation	anti-inflammatory drugs (ibuprofen)
	opioids (such as fentanyl, morphine)
Control anxiety	benzodiazepines (such as midazolam, or Versed)
Control stomach acid production	antihistamine agents (such as Pepcid)

are permitting as they sign anesthetic consent forms. In days long past, there was a prevailing attitude of paternalism: "the doctor knows best." Over time this attitude has yielded to the desire by many patients to have more information.

Most people understand that adverse events can occur in surgery and anesthesia. If complications ensue, patients are more accepting if they have been previously informed about the possibilities. On the other hand, if they have never been informed of the risk of an adverse outcome, such as the loss of a tooth, a vocal cord injury, or a heart attack, patients are less tolerant, and sometimes—understandably— very upset. Since anesthesia is an inescapable part of most surgeries, patients have a tendency to provide consent as a matter of course rather than having a candid discussion with the anesthesiologist. This discussion, however, emphasizing risks and safeguards, is an essential part of obtaining valid consent to proceed with the anesthetic.

Early on during your interview, preparations will be made for inserting an intravenous catheter, or IV (table 3.3). This is an anxiety-provoking time for adult patients whose veins are small or tortuous or for younger patients, who appear to be more sensitive to pain and to the psychological stresses of having a needlestick. An IV insertion can be made less uncomfortable if it is preceded by a small injection of local anesthetic in the skin. This local anesthetic stings briefly but reduces the pain of inserting the larger IV catheter, especially if it does not easily enter the vein. If you are very sensitive or anxious, an anesthetizing cream can be placed over the likely IV placement

Table 3.3 **Preparing a patient for anesthesia**

Performing preoperative evaluation and medication administration

Placing intravenous (IV) catheter and fluid infusion

Administering sedation to reduce anxiety

Placing of nerve blocks and/or invasive monitoring devices

Transporting to operating room

Moving to OR bed

Making sure patient is comfortable, with no undue pressure or stretching of body parts

Adding bolsters or padding as necessary over pressure points site forty-five minutes before insertion, which effectively numbs the skin. It is preferable for the patient to be lying down, or at least reclining, during IV insertion because sometimes people faint, often unpredictably, due to a reflex drop in blood pressure and heart rate. Even the strongest or toughest individual may faint; it is not necessarily related to fear or anxiety. After the catheter is placed in a vein, an electrolyte solution is infused through the catheter to replace fluid deficits from the long fasting period that most patients experience before they come to the operating room.

Since a surgical patient may be anxious or unsettled as he or she awaits the trip to the operating room, the next step is to provide a degree of preoperative sedation. This sedation is not given until consent has been obtained for both the anesthesia and the surgery because patients must be alert to give informed consent. Sedation is usually initiated with a benzodiazepine, a drug in the Valium family, and sometimes with an opioid, a medication in the morphine family. Most patients feel very pleasant effects as sedation is administered. If you become somnolent after sedation, anesthesia personnel will usually provide oxygen as well as cardiac and oxygenation monitors to ensure safety, continually attending to you until the operation has begun. Once all of this is accomplished, you will be escorted to the operating room.

Depending on circumstances, you may be visited by your surgeon in the preoperative holding area, or you may be greeted by him or her in the operating room as preparations are made to begin anesthesia. In the operating room, you will be asked to transfer from the carriage or stretcher to a narrow operating table. A flurry of activity will ensue, as the anesthesia team and the operating room nurses get you ready for surgery and ensure your safety. Many patients have no memory of any of this because they have received sedative medications, even though they may have been alert and conversant during this period.

From the anesthesia standpoint, safety measures are paramount as soon as care is initiated (table 3.4). Once you are on the operating room table, several monitors will be attached to you. Electrocardiographic (EKG) leads are placed on the chest to monitor heart function and rhythm. An automatic blood pressure cuff is placed on one of your arms to measure blood pressure intermittently throughout the surgery. A pulse oximeter, a small clip or adhesive tape with a light sensor, is placed on a finger or thumb to measure oxygen levels continuously. Other monitors are in common use, including temperature monitoring and measurement of carbon dioxide coming from the lungs, to ensure adequate ventilation throughout. The

Table 3.4 The steps for initiation (induction) of general anesthesia

Administering preoperative sedation (optional; not all patients require sedation)

Placing monitors

Providing preoxygenation with face mask (ensuring adequate reservoir of oxygen in lungs)

Infusing induction drug to cause loss of consciousness

Applying face-mask ventilation (after patient stops breathing)

Administering muscle relaxant agent (not necessary for all types of induction)

Placing breathing tube

temperature and carbon dioxide monitors are usually initiated after anesthesia has begun. (See pages 30–33 for illustrations of these monitors.)

During the placement of your monitors (all of which will feel as if they have been in a refrigerator somewhere), oxygen will be administered. This is an important safety issue because filling the lungs with oxygen allows considerable time to place an airway device after you go "off to sleep" and slow or cease your breathing efforts (see below). While you are still conscious, you will usually be asked if you are in a comfortable position, and efforts will be made to pad any joint or skin surface that might be subjected to unusual pressure or impact.

After these steps have been completed, a syringe of medication will be injected into the IV, and within twenty or so seconds you will be unconscious. These intravenous medications, the prototype of which is sodium thiopental, or Pentothal, rapidly lead to unconsciousness and are generally quite pleasant to experience, although they may initially irritate the vein, causing a brief burning sensation. For the past decade, propofol has been the agent most commonly used to initiate anesthesia in adults because it is cleared from the body rapidly and tends to suppress nausea and vomiting.

The profound unconsciousness that constitutes general anesthesia is very deep indeed. This is far beyond what most people think of as "going to sleep," for which we can all be grateful. You certainly would not tolerate a surgeon coming into your room at night to make an incision into your skin, no matter how deeply you were sleeping. The expression "going to sleep" to describe anesthesia is thus a poor characterization of what actually occurs.

Naturally, patients worry quite a bit about being aware of surgery or pain while under anesthesia, and this concern has been heightened by reports of such phenomena on television in the past decade. While this is possible, it is very unusual. The ability to recall events that have occurred while under anesthesia have been reported to occur in 1 to 3 percent of cases. There is some evidence that well-anesthetized patients may actually have the ability to successfully recall some verbal cues given to them while unconscious. However, this does not translate into the ability to be awake, sense pain or unpleasant emotions, or recall these things in the postoperative period. This sort of dreadful outcome is rare. There are ways to protect patients from this outcome: brain wave monitors derived from electroencephalographic (EEG) activity and other types of cerebral monitors are under development. These monitors allow an assessment of the "depth" of anesthesia, to ensure that the patient is not aware while undergoing surgery.

For many years a patient's vital signs were taken as evidence of the depth of anesthesia; however, these parameters are not reliable indicators of what a patient may be experiencing. Hence, there has been increasing interest in the profession in monitors for brain activity. As with all medical devices, these new brain monitors have drawbacks and insufficiencies. But the instruments allow more confidence on the part of the anesthesiologist, particularly when a patient may not be able to tolerate usual amounts of anesthetic drugs, such as patients in shock, patients with severe trauma, patients undergoing cardiac surgery, and women in labor requiring emergency cesarean sections. Still, there is controversy about the use of these monitors. Recent trials comparing the risk of awareness among hundreds of patients under general anesthesia have not uniformly found the devices to be protective. While potentially useful as a component of monitoring, these monitors are clearly not foolproof, and the search for more accurate sensors continues.

The drugs used for the initiation, or *induction*, of anesthesia in adults, delivered through an IV, produce various effects—some of them desirable, some not. After such a drug is administered, the patient's speech becomes slurred and then ceases. The eyelids close in most cases, and the lines of the face relax and soften. The patient does indeed appear to have gone rapidly to sleep. However, profound changes in the vital systems also occur. Breathing usually ceases, blood pressure typically drops significantly, and the heart rate may either drop or quicken, depending on the drug administered and the patient's state of excitation.

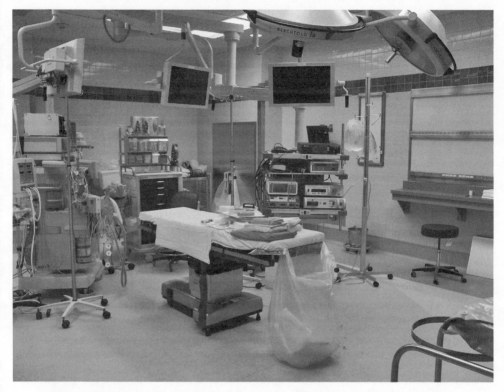

Figure 3.1 The inside of an operating room. A complex array of anesthesia implements and monitors, tools for orthopedic surgery, and imaging screens and cameras for minimally invasive procedures require a large amount of space.

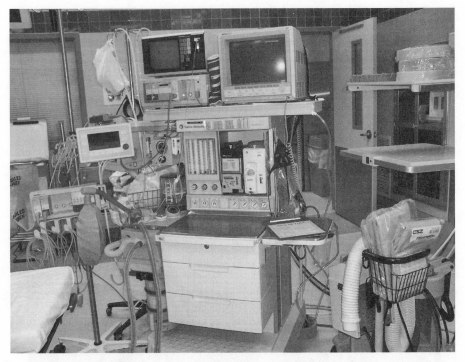

Figure 3.2 The modern anesthesia machine not only delivers gases with precision, but also has a built-in mechanical ventilator as well as many monitors and safeguards to help ensure patient safety. The newest generation of machines presents nearly all relevant data on a touch screen, which allows ventilation and gas flows and mixtures to be adjusted. On such machines, the knobs for titrating gases have been eliminated.

Figure 3.3 (facing, top) The patient is being readied for anesthesia. Monitors for automated blood pressure detection and electrocardiography (EKG) have been placed on the arm and chest. On one of the fingers or thumb, a pulse oximetry probe will be placed for continuous monitoring of blood oxygen content. After induction of anesthesia, the patient's temperature and exhaled carbon dioxide will also be monitored.

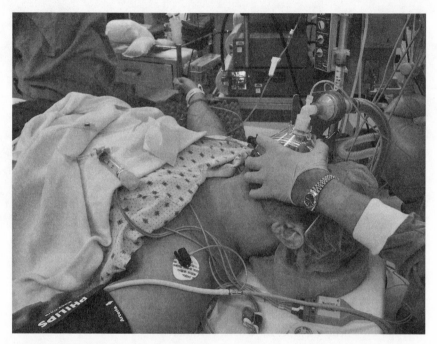

Figure 3.4 Just before the drugs for induction of anesthesia are injected, the patient breathes pure oxygen for several minutes. This process, termed *preoxygenation*, ensures maximum lung and blood oxygen content, providing a reserve for the period when the tracheal tube is placed in the airway. As soon as consciousness is lost, ventilation with oxygen is provided using the face mask and the anesthesia bag on the machine, until complete relaxation occurs. If placing the artificial airway turns out to be difficult and requires more time than expected, this reservoir of oxygen in the lungs helps maintain blood oxygen at acceptable levels for much longer than if the patient had simply been breathing room air before induction.

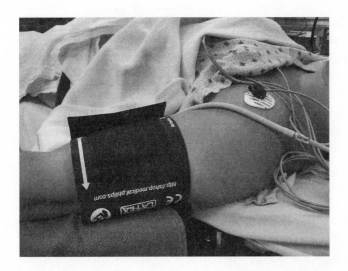

Figure 3.5 After the anesthesia induction drugs are injected, patients rapidly become unconscious and relaxed. When this is achieved, the face mask is removed and a laryngoscope is used to retract the tongue and soft tissues as the anesthetist peers into the throat. Once the *glottis*, or opening to the airway, is visualized, the tracheal tube is placed. In some cases of general anesthesia, a tracheal tube is not necessary, and instead a soft mask at the end of a shorter tube, called a *laryngeal mask airway*, is inserted to prevent the tongue from falling back to block the airway. Either of these implements permits connecting the patient's airway to the anesthesia machine via a series of flexible tubes called the *circuit*. Administration of anesthetic gases as well as the desired concentration of oxygen then begins.

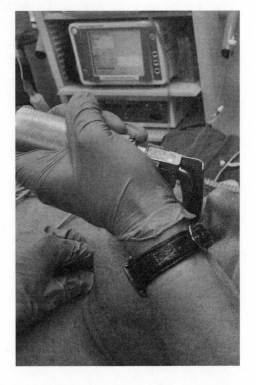

Because the patient is not getting adequate ventilation in this state, the anesthesiologist must intervene. Oxygen must be reliably delivered to the lungs or the patient will suffer severe injury. This is seldom challenging and usually involves initially ventilating the patient with a face mask, followed by inserting a tube to carry gases to the lungs throughout the time under anesthesia. These gases include life-sustaining oxygen and potent vapors that frequently form the foundation of the anesthetic. The tube that is inserted into the throat may be a tracheal tube, placed through the voice box with an instrument that lights the back of the throat, called a laryngoscope. Or, it may be a laryngeal mask (LMA), which sits at the back of the tongue, over the opening to the voice box.

The LMA has become increasingly popular in recent years because it is simpler to insert for the anesthesiologist and less traumatic to patients. The mask appears to cause less postoperative sore throat than endotracheal tubes and less noxious stimulation to the patient and to his or her vital signs at the time of placement. For various reasons, such as full stomach or gastroesophageal reflux (heartburn), these laryngeal mask devices are not appropriate for all patients. Before the introduction of the LMA, in the late 1980s, shorter surgical cases were frequently managed by placement of a face mask on the patient, while the anesthesiologist or nurse anesthetist worked hard to maintain an adequate seal to the face. Gas delivery and ventilation throughout the surgery depended on the integrity of the fit between this mask and the patient's face. The LMA has vastly simplified this process, allowing the medical personnel to pay attention to many other tasks during the surgical case.

After the breathing tube is secured and its position is confirmed, surgical preparation will begin. This includes scrubbing your skin with antiseptic and placing sterile drapes. Immediately after induction, the anesthesiologist or nurse anesthetist will begin to administer a *maintenance* anesthetic, which involves delivering drugs for amnesia, unconsciousness, and pain control for the duration of the surgery (table 3.5). The maintenance anesthetic may comprise gases alone, known as *inhalation anesthesia*, or intravenous drugs alone, referred to as *total intravenous anesthesia*. Commonly, a combination of both anesthetic vapors and intravenous agents are administered to ensure that the various goals of a general anesthetic are accomplished.

Whether an anesthetic lasts for ten minutes or ten hours, the emphasis is on vigilance. Respiratory difficulties, bleeding, heart dysfunction, or allergic reactions can occur at any time of the anesthetic, including the

Table 3.5 Drugs and agents to maintain anesthesia

Drugs	Examples
Volatile gases	halogenated hydrocarbons, such as isoflurane
Propofol infusion	given by constant drip
Nitrous oxide	a very weak anesthetic gas, with good pain relief properties, that usually accompanies propofol or volatile gas
Opioid drugs	derivatives of morphine, to provide depth of anesthesia and ensure pain control
Muscle relaxants	if needed for the surgical procedure; typically for abdominal, pelvic, thoracic, heart, brain, or major head/neck surgery

induction period, maintenance phase, or emergence from anesthesia. As with the takeoff and landing of airline flights, the beginning and end of the anesthetic are most critical and hazardous. Throughout the anesthetic, vital signs are recorded, monitors are scanned, and vital functions are assessed continuously. The anesthetist or anesthesiologist has many tools for addressing any problems that arise, from treating high or low blood pressure with appropriate medications, to suctioning the airway, to using drugs that relax the bronchial tubes in order to improve the flow of oxygen and gases through them.

When the surgeon notifies the nurse anesthetist or anesthesiologist that the case is nearly at its completion, the anesthetics will be reduced and then turned off. The goal is for you to recover your airway reflexes, resume spontaneous breathing, and maintain a stable blood pressure, as well as achieve mental alertness, as smoothly and quickly as possible (table 3.6). Adequate relief of your pain is crucial. To suddenly stop anesthesia after a large incision has been made, without the benefit of pain-control medications or techniques, is the equivalent of awakening in the morning after a night of liberal alcohol consumption accompanied by a serious injury—you would suddenly awaken to severe discomfort.

To avoid this outcome, pain therapies such as IV opioid medications (the morphine family of drugs), IV anti-inflammatory medications, and injection of local anesthetics to numb the surgical incision site are given before the anesthetic is completely discontinued. In fact, pain medications

Table 3.6 When the patient awakens from anesthesia

Discontinuation of maintenance phase agents

Resumption of spontaneous breathing (with adequate lung function)

Evidence of return of airway reflexes (cough, gag reflexes)

Stabilized blood pressure and cardiac function

Adequate levels of bloodstream oxygenation

Return of adequate muscle strength (for strong cough, head lift, extremity motion)

Wakefulness and alertness

---

actively contribute to, and deepen, the level of anesthesia in some beneficial ways aside from mere pain relief. Opioid medications are components of virtually every general anesthetic provided for a procedure that is expected to cause pain.

As you begin to show signs of awakening, preparations are made for emergence from anesthesia. The airway is suctioned to remove any secretions from your throat so that you do not inhale them when the airway tube is removed. Soon, you will begin to respond to verbal commands and demonstrate purposeful behavior. Before the breathing tube is removed, your ability to breathe easily and to cough is assessed, as well as whether you have recovered muscle strength. Although you will show initial signs of being alert at this stage, few patients remember any of this because the mind is still somewhat clouded by anesthetics. Monitors are then removed, and you will be helped to a stretcher and transported to the PACU. The anesthesia provider remains in close attendance during this period, vigilant for any complications, particularly breathing difficulties.

On arrival in PACU, most patients are alert enough to begin to appreciate their surroundings. Monitors are once again applied, as is oxygen. The anesthesiologist or anesthetist will take note of the new vital signs, ensuring stability, and then discuss the patient's care with the PACU nurse who is assuming responsibility. This detailed turnover is crucial to help the nurse understand any concerns or problems that may have arisen in the operating room, as well as those to be expected from the type of surgical procedure, the background of the patient, and the anesthesia medications that were administered.

There are several goals for you during the PACU period, such as ensuring the stability of your cardiovascular and respiratory systems. You should be alert enough to communicate your feelings and needs. Any surgical issues, such as drains or bleeding, are noted and followed. Orders are generally given to administer medications to control pain and nausea. These are administered at the discretion of the PACU nurse, and such orders usually include parameters for when the anesthesia or surgical team need to be called for consultation. Scoring systems are in widespread use to achieve a standard among facilities as to when the patient is adequately recovered and ready to be taken to the hospital room or to the next level of recovery.

If you are slated to return home on the day of surgery, a step-down or second-phase recovery experience is usually next. You may be moved to another unit, or there may simply be a reduction in the intensity of nursing care and attention while you remain in one place. Either way, the requirements are different from those in the initial recovery period. The purpose of this second phase is to ensure that patients are "street fit," that is, able to function at home without skilled nursing care. The patient must be able to ambulate (or use crutches after leg surgeries) and must be free from significant nausea. All vital signs must be stable, pain must be manageable with oral pain medications, and a competent adult must be available into whose care the patient can be discharged.

From the initiation of the first medication until delivery into the recovery area, anesthesia care is all about vigilance, safety, and control of adverse influences related to surgery and the anesthetics themselves. During general anesthesia, deep planes of unconsciousness require airway protection and assistance with ventilation for most patients. Multiple agents are usually combined to provide the desirable aspects of a general anesthetic; today these agents are much more effective and less noxious than anesthetic agents used in the past. Still, nagging side effects persist, particularly postoperative nausea and inadequate pain control after invasive or extensive surgery. This is especially true when general anesthesia and opioid medications are used, without other specific efforts to reduce postoperative pain.

General anesthesia has been a wondrous addition to the medical armamentarium, and administering it has become the dedicated goal of an entire field of medicine. Many improvements in anesthesia patient safety have been made since the early days of inhaling ether from a cloth held under

Table 3.7 **Common side effects of general anesthesia**

Side effect	Frequency
Nausea and vomiting	10 to 60% (depending on surgical type; patient population)
Drowsiness or dizziness	At least 50%
Pain at the surgical site	Virtually all
Sore throat	10 to 50%

the nose. In the past two decades, there has been a further reduction in severe adverse events and mortality attributable solely to anesthesia.

However, there is no question that, despite its advantages, general anesthesia has limitations and drawbacks too (table 3.7). If you have had a procedure under general anesthesia, or have cared for a loved one emerging from general anesthesia, you will be able to relate to the common aftereffects of the brain-altering medications. Postoperative nausea and vomiting is a frequent problem. Depending on the study site, the population under investigation, the type of surgery, and the anesthetic agents delivered, it affects between 10 and 60 percent of patients.

Untold dollars and research studies have been brought to bear on postoperative nausea, called the "big little problem" of anesthesia. Although nausea is not life threatening, patients have made it clear that it is most unpleasant. Many relate that they would pay out-of-pocket for assurance that their procedure would not be followed by nausea or vomiting. When surveyed, surgical candidates frequently place nausea at the top of the list of the most undesirable perioperative occurrences. This will not be surprising to you if you have spent a day or so after anesthesia lying prostrate, unable to function because of this misery.

The agents of modern anesthesia are certainly an improvement on those used by previous generations of anesthesiologists, such as chloroform, ether, and cyclopropane. The new agents cause less nausea and provide better control of the anesthetic itself. Anesthetic gases that leave the body quickly, such as desflurane and sevoflurane, and those with intrinsic antinausea properties, such as propofol, all represent real advances. Furthermore, effective classes of antinausea drugs and anesthetic techniques that can reduce nausea have been developed. At most institutions, prophylactic antinausea drugs such as ondansetron (Zofran) are administered as a matter of course during the anesthetic. Their effectiveness in patients at significant risk of nausea is indisputable. In patients at very high risk—those with a strong history of postoperative nausea or severe motion sickness—applying a topical patch of scopolamine, often used for motion sickness, can be effective.

Even with these management techniques, the possibility of postoperative nausea and vomiting persists. For some patients, due to the length or type of surgery, or a minimal need for nausea-producing opioids, the risk of postoperative nausea is low. In such circumstances, the anesthesiologist may opt to "wait and see," treating nausea if it occurs in the postoperative period, rather than providing prophylactic medications in the OR.

The feeling of an anesthesia "hangover," a combination of drowsiness, dizziness, and confusion, is also a common complaint. Many patients characterize this prolonged effect as "taking a long time to wake up," even though they can carry on a conversation during this period. These symptoms often become true delirium in the elderly, whose brains are susceptible to changes of many kinds. Once again, shorter-acting agents tend to allow return to a feeling of normalcy sooner than with previous generations of anesthetics. These agents make possible today's shorter hospital stays after surgery.

Contributing to the anesthesia-related dysphoria that you may have after surgery are the medications typically administered to provide pain relief so that you may wake up with a reasonable degree of pain control. Pain medications, usually opioids (the derivatives of morphine, such as fentanyl, meperidine, and hydromorphone), are generally administered before, during, and after surgery as part of the anesthetic. These medications are effective in controlling pain because they bind to certain brain and spinal cord receptors. They allow a reasonably comfortable transition from unconsciousness to an alert state when the surgery involves an extensive incision. Unfortunately, these agents also produce a host of adverse side effects, including ongoing sleepiness, nausea, dizziness, respiratory depression, itching, and constipation. Various techniques are available to the anesthesiologist and surgeon to reduce your need for opioids, such as substituting anti-inflammatory agents for these medications, or injecting local anesthetic drugs into the site of the surgical wound.

Some patients who undergo surgery with general anesthesia awaken with considerable discomfort, despite the liberal use of opioids and other pain medications. Different people have different pain thresholds: it is estimated that required opioid doses for relief of pain from a surgical stimulus can vary tenfold from one person to another! Some types of surgery are extremely painful, and side effects such as sedation limit the amount of opioid pain medication that a patient may receive. Pain ranges from unpleasant to intolerable, and substantial numbers of patients continue to suffer from pain while hospitalized for medical or surgical conditions. Many ambulatory surgical patients have pain that is moderate to severe on the day after surgery.

Pain is not only a source of patient discomfort; it is also a cause of a physiological stress response that, if unchecked, can have important consequences for the body. For this reason, effectively controlling pain is an essential task for all physicians, especially anesthesiologists. In addition to the measures mentioned above, regional anesthesia techniques, which employ local anesthetics in the spine or at the site of peripheral nerves, are essential tools of the anesthesiologist. (I explore these techniques in detail in later chapters.)

There are other adverse effects of general anesthesia. Because of poor ventilation during profound degrees of unconsciousness, the patient's airway is generally secured with a tube placed at the back of the tongue or in the throat. The widespread use of these tubes means that sore throat is a frequent postoperative complaint. Ten to 50 percent of patients will complain of hoarseness, scratchiness, or pain in the throat after a general anesthetic involving a tracheal tube. Since the newer form of breathing tube, the LMA, fits over the voice box, it allows the patient to breathe on his or her own while avoiding obstruction of ventilation from a relaxed tongue or soft palate. These devices work well and seem to cause less sore throat in patients for whom they are appropriate.

These, then, are the most common side effects of general anesthesia. There are, in addition, outcomes of general anesthesia that are unexpected and unusual. They affect a small fraction of patients who undergo anesthesia. These rare adverse outcomes are explored in the next chapter.

Chapter 4
Complications, Risk Assessment, and Safety

 How do physicians assess patient risk before anesthesia and surgery?

Who is at the highest risk for complications during general anesthesia?

How has safety in anesthesia evolved in recent years?

What are the most common complications of general anesthesia?

How often do these complications occur?

How can I be protected from such complications?

What happens when controlling the airway is difficult during anesthesia?

What causes the most complications in the operating room?

Assessing risk in patients who undergo any medical procedure is an exercise in epidemiology, which is the study of the incidence of disease (or in this case, adverse outcomes) in a population. Physicians learn little about overall risk by simply observing one or a few cases, so studies usually assess a treatment's effect on a population or group rather than on a few individuals. Studying small numbers of people can create bias, and although reports of individual cases do affect physician practice patterns, large clinical trials are much more valuable. Physicians must be cautious, however, in applying the results of large trials to individual patients. If the circumstances and patient characteristics described in the study are not exactly the same as those affecting the individual, then the results may not be applicable. Nonetheless, the large, randomized, clinical trial is the best tool that physicians have to help them understand the result of different types of treatments and learn safety and risk information so that they can provide the best care possible for their patients.

Medical professionals often create risk-scoring systems to help predict outcomes for patients. These systems usually involve assigning points for certain traits or conditions, which are then tallied and compared to a benchmark to predict the likelihood of adverse events based on epidemiological studies. Often these scoring systems conflict with each other, and they can be frustratingly complex. Fortunately, in anesthesia, the most commonly used system is rather simple, and despite much more complex alternatives, this system has served the profession well. Anesthesiologists assign patient risk levels according to the following physical status (PS) scoring system:

PS 1: A healthy patient with no conditions that affect anesthesia risk.

PS 2: A patient with one or more well-controlled systemic diseases. The increase in risk for surgery and anesthesia is minimal.

PS 3: A patient with poorly managed systemic disease or disease that has progressed to end-organ damage, increasing the risk of anesthesia.

PS 4: An unstable patient with a disease or condition that represents a constant threat to life. The risk of anesthesia and surgery is very high.

PS 5: A patient who is not expected to survive through a surgical procedure.

PS 6: A patient who is an organ donor.

Within this scoring system, emergency procedures are identified with an "E" after the number. Extra risk is attributed to any emergency case because there is little time for physicians to prepare the patients, and they often arrive with a full stomach, which increases the risks of anesthesia. Most patients are assigned to the PS 1 or 2 categories, with very few in the PS 4 or 5 categories.

This system provides an overall index of a patient's risk during anesthesia and surgery without unnecessary and complicating detail. Each patient who undergoes anesthesia in the United States is assigned a physical status score. This score allows effective communication among clinicians, assists with appropriate billing (very sick patients require much more resources and time), and facilitates the review of cases and complications for quality improvement exercises.

✦ Most of the preoperative risk assessment, like any medical diagnostic process, is derived from the history and physical examination performed by your anesthesiologist at the bedside. The knowledge that your anesthesiologist gains from discussing with you medical problems and prior anesthetic experiences is far more valuable to him or her than the results of several nonspecific tests.

Twenty years ago, a healthy 30-year-old patient reporting for a minor surgery, such as a knee arthroscopy, would have received hundreds of dollars worth of testing, including blood chemistries, blood counts, chest x-ray, and probably an electrocardiogram—all of them essentially worthless to the care of the patient in the operating room. Physicians have since learned that the most useful information is gathered at the bedside, in discussions with the patient, and while performing a physical exam. They can use this information to order specific laboratory tests that focus on abnormalities that are uncovered in your history and physical (table 4.1). Today, most healthy patients undergoing a minor or moderately invasive surgical procedure require no lab tests preoperatively. Some studies suggest that elderly people may benefit from a routine electrocardiogram, but even this is debatable if no abnormalities are apparent in the history or physical exam. This change in routine preoperative testing reduces health care expenditures by billions of dollars annually, while saving individual patients time, inconvenience, and discomfort.

One of the most crucial aspects of preoperative evaluation is cardiac testing. Complications related to the cardiovascular system, although very uncommon in low-risk patients, are among the most debilitating of the serious complications that patients may experience during or after surgery. Predicting such complications as myocardial infarction (heart attack), cardiac arrest, and heart rhythm disturbances has proved challenging. Physicians must avoid unnecessary testing because it may involve invasive procedures with additional inherent risk. Furthermore, *false positives* may occur, in which patients may be subjected needlessly to further testing or procedures, with all the wasted time, effort, and money that this process entails.

The patchwork of practices and recommendations for preoperative car-

Table 4.1 **Common laboratory tests before surgery**

Test	Purpose	Relevant condition
Blood count (CBC)	Evaluate adequacy of red blood cells	Anemia
Blood glucose	Determine "sugar" level in blood	Diabetes
Chest x-ray	Evaluate chest conditions	Lung disease, heart failure
Electrocardiogram	Assessment of heart	Coronary artery disease, heart rhythm disturbances
Electrolytes	Evaluate potassium, sodium in blood	Taking diuretic drugs
Urea nitrogen/ creatinine levels	Assessment of kidney function	Chronic kidney disease

diac testing that existed ten to twenty years ago was insufficient and incon-sistent. After hearing your medical history, one physician might consider you stable for surgery, whereas another would cancel the procedure and send you for testing to evaluate your heart. In the mid-1990s, a committee of anesthesiologists, internists, and cardiologists developed recommenda-tions for physicians to promote consistency, reduce waste, and avoid test-related complications for patients. These experts examined hundreds of studies on the utility of various tests that physicians used to predict opera-tive cardiac risk and developed a set of recommendations for preoperative cardiac testing known as the American College of Cardiology / American Heart Association guidelines. This decision-making tool is based on three essential elements: a patient's history, his or her ability to exercise, and the invasiveness of the planned surgery. Using these three pieces of informa-tion, a physician can determine whether a patient slated for surgery will benefit from preoperative testing or can simply go straight to the operating room with appropriate monitoring.

Although other cardiac risk assessment tools exist, this scheme is most commonly used today. A central tenet of these guidelines is that the process of testing patients and correcting their underlying problems should be less risky to patients than having them simply undergo the planned surgery without these interventions. In patients known to have stable coronary heart disease, recent studies appear to favor going forward with the surgery, as opposed to engaging in cardiac evaluation and invasive therapy.

Diseases of other organ systems besides the heart can significantly increase operative risk, and these also require close attention by your anesthesiologist in the preoperative period. Prominent among these are obstructive lung diseases (such as asthma and emphysema), liver and kidney insufficiency, poorly controlled diabetes, muscle diseases, and bleeding abnormalities. Patients with vascular diseases, such as stroke or occlusive arterial disease, are at significant risk for heart attack in the period immediately after an operation, especially if undergoing a vascular surgery procedure.

A thorough preoperative evaluation coupled with an appropriate anesthetic plan for the period during and immediately after surgery is necessary to ensure patient safety. Whatever the nature of your underlying disease, it is the anesthesiologist's responsibility to ensure that your medical conditions have been optimized before coming to the operating room. If not, it may be possible to initiate or improve therapies at the bedside right before the operation. In some cases, however, there is no choice but to delay the surgery until more intensive or appropriate therapy is begun or continued in consultation with your primary care provider or a specialist.

The specifics of your medical history are not the only detail anesthesiologists use when determining your overall surgical risk. Even the most ill or medically unstable patient may be able to tolerate a short, painless procedure. The invasiveness and duration of the surgical procedure are also important aspects of perioperative risk. The lowest tier of surgical risk involves short, nonstimulating procedures with minimal tissue trauma, such as removal of skin lesions, cataract surgery, or surgery on the fingers or toes. A more moderate level of surgical risk includes the majority of common surgical procedures, such as gall bladder removal, hip or knee surgery, or ear, nose, and throat procedures. Prostate surgery and gynecological surgeries are also associated with moderate levels of risk. The procedures that seem to involve the highest degree of risk are those that are quite invasive, such as heart or aortic surgery; those that involve significant blood loss or fluid shifts; and those that are performed as emergency surgery. Vascular surgery on clogged arteries falls in this category as well, probably because of its long duration and the well-known underlying heart disease that afflicts most of these patients.

Anesthesiologists must assess the risks of surgical cases by integrating information about patients and their diseases, patients' functional capacity, and the nature of the procedures they undergo. The next step is to modify and manage these risks in the best way possible to obtain a favorable outcome. There are several interventions that may be used to reduce these risks. In some cases, you may have to cancel or delay your surgery until you receive additional treatment in the inpatient or outpatient setting. For instance, a patient with angina whose chest pains have been getting worse or have been occurring at rest should not undergo elective surgery until the reason for this deterioration in heart function is discovered and addressed. The risk of a heart attack in the perioperative period for such a patient is quite high, and he or she should not undergo surgery except in an emergency situation. In patients with other types of disease, physicians may deliver therapy in the immediate preoperative period to reduce risk and ensure control of the underlying process. Fortunately, many patients with significant underlying diseases are evaluated and treated by their own doctors before coming to the operating room, so cancellation is much less common than it used to be. Furthermore, anesthesiologists now perform preoperative screening by phone and computer, or in a preoperative clinic.

Physicians can reduce your risk of complications during a planned procedure in many ways. Preoperative medications may be administered to reduce acid reflux, prevent a flare-up of asthma or emphysema, reduce the chance of thyroid hyperactivity, prevent blood pressure elevations, or protect against several other issues. One of the most important interventions that your anesthesiologist can provide before, during, and after your surgery is the administration of a group of medications called beta-receptor blockers. These medications protect the heart in patients with known coronary heart disease (blockages of the vessels that supply blood to the heart itself) and have been shown in many studies to reduce mortality for this high-risk population. Note, however, that a recent large, prospective trial has cast a doubt on how effective these drugs are when applied to all at-risk patients. Certain subsets of patients may particularly benefit from these drugs, and efforts are ongoing to define these specific groups.

Monitoring is an important aspect of patient safety and has undergone substantial modification in the last decade. If you receive anesthesia, you will be attached to various machines that continuously display vital health parameters. These invariably include the electrocardiogram leads, an automated blood pressure cuff, and pulse oximetry, which uses light absorption by a finger or earlobe to determine oxygen levels in the bloodstream. These three monitors are used throughout hospitals for any invasive procedure that requires sedation and therefore alters your consciousness level.

Additional monitors placed on you in the operating room include sensors for temperature and carbon dioxide monitoring. The carbon dioxide monitor provides second-to-second evidence of ongoing breathing and has recently become a standard of monitoring in anesthesia. It is used to confirm that the breathing tube was placed correctly in patients under general anesthesia and to show the ongoing adequacy of ventilation. Carbon dioxide monitoring and pulse oximetry, along with improved medical skills and knowledge, are the most likely reasons for the significant reduction in death or brain injuries from failures of airway management during anesthetics in recent years. In prior generations, airway management difficulty was a major cause of adverse patient outcomes related to anesthesia.

Anesthesiology is an atypical medical specialty in that it is usually not involved in direct diagnosis and long-term treatment of disease, as most specialties are (including pain management, a subspecialty of anesthesiology). Rather, it involves caring for you, the surgical patient, while you are involved in the surgical process, treating your medical problems in the period surrounding your surgery, and ensuring that you receive effective pain management. The pharmacological agents that produce anesthesia result in various alterations of your vital systems, which may adversely interact with underlying diseases. In addition, the consequences of surgical trauma may affect you in ways that anesthesiologists must interpret and treat.

Because anesthesia imposes risks on patients, patient safety has always been a centerpiece of anesthesia care. The goal of anesthesiologists is to arrive in the recovery room with a patient who is as healthy and functional as he or she was preoperatively, at least as far as is possible given the surgery. This paradigm mandates that patient safety is always the first consideration in anesthesia.

Large-scale studies of anesthesia practice in the past decade have established an anesthetic mortality rate somewhere between 1 in 30,000 and 1 in 100,000, depending on the definition used for death "related" to anesthesia. Deaths that are clearly attributable to preventable anesthesia mishaps approximate 1 in 100,000. This is a far cry from the middle of the twentieth century, when anesthesia was widely considered to be extremely dangerous. Today, patient death in the perioperative period is more likely to result from surgical complications or from the response of an underlying disease to the surgical or anesthetic process than directly from the anesthetic interventions the patient received. This is a testimony to the dramatic improvement in safety that anesthesiologists have witnessed over the past several decades.

Several organizations are responsible for making your safety in the operating room a continual focus of health care professionals. The American Society of Anesthesiologists and the American Association of Nurse Anesthetists promulgate practice guidelines to help ensure patient safety, and they continue to develop these guidelines as new information becomes available. Research foundations, such as the Foundation for Anesthesia Education and Research, provide supportive grants to promising young investigators who develop new anesthetic techniques, monitoring systems, and medications to advance the cause of safe anesthesia. The Anesthesia Patient Safety Foundation (APSF), founded in the mid-twentieth century, is a venerable organization whose sole purpose is to minimize the risks of anesthesia to patients. This foundation participates in policy development, awards grants for safety-related research, and educates practitioners in the area of patient protection in the perioperative period. APSF has participated in the development of the National Patient Safety Center, an organization concerned with the protection of patients in all areas of medicine.

Despite the emphasis on safety, complications related to the administration of anesthesia continue to exist. To some extent, this is probably unavoidable, given the stresses and trauma that patients undergo in the perioperative period, as well as the profound impact that anesthetic drugs have on multiple organ systems. It is important to make a distinction between side effects and complications of anesthesia, which are both adverse effects of treatment. Side effects are common adverse effects that you experience because of drugs or medical techniques, and although they are undesirable, they are largely unavoidable. Side effects are undoubtedly unpleasant for you, but they do not generally cause any significant injury. Complications are much less common than side effects after a treatment or procedure but are more severe, resulting in patient injury or an escalation of care (such as transfer to the intensive care unit or blood transfusion). However, there can be overlap between types of side effects and complications: for example, mild nausea is widely considered a side effect of anesthesia, whereas severe postoperative nausea with vomiting, necessitating hospital admission and multiple doses of drugs, could be viewed as a complication.

Several fairly common side effects of anesthesia were discussed in chapter 3. In this chapter, I explore the potential complications of anesthesia (table 4.2). Despite the rarity of most complications, they occur with frustrating regularity over time in a busy anesthesia practice. The analysis of cause and effect, with attempts at subsequent process improvement, is an

Table 4.2 Possible severe complications of general anesthesia

Major allergic response (affecting breathing and/or blood pressure)

Malignant hyperthermia

Corneal abrasion

Loss of vision

Larynx injury (such as cartilage dislocation)

Hoarseness due to vocal cord paralysis

Brain or heart injury resulting from difficulty in placing or inability to place breathing tube

Aspiration of stomach contents into airway and lungs (pulmonary aspiration)

Blood pressure disturbances

Heart attack or cardiac arrest

Stroke

Postoperative confusion (cognitive dysfunction)

Death

essential part of improving any type of health care, including the delivery of anesthesia and surgical services.

If you are unfamiliar with anesthesia, you may find yourself fearing the possibility of "dying on the table." Fortunately, the safety of general anesthesia has improved dramatically in the past half a century, and death caused by general or regional anesthesia in healthy patients is extremely unusual, as noted above. Anesthetic mortalities, though they are rare, usually occur in patients with substantial perioperative risk related to heart, lung, brain, or vascular diseases. Because of the intensity of monitoring and the safety of modern anesthesia equipment and drugs, it is probably true that you take a bigger risk by going for a ride in your car than by having general anesthesia. This analogy is often used at the bedside in the preoperative discussion to allay patient anxieties. However, other risks of general anesthesia are not quite so rare. Severe reactions to a medication administered for the purpose of anesthesia, or the antibiotics universally given to reduce surgical infections, are likely to occur in approximately 1 in 6,000 cases. These responses can occur even if you have been exposed to the same medications before, although this does make the possibility less likely.

The expression of these allergic or allergic-type reactions is quite variable. Mild allergic reactions, such as a transient skin rash or brief drop in blood pressure, could be missed entirely. Severe reactions, however, may result in life-threatening blood pressure depression, difficulty with ventilation, or even cardiac arrest. Because so many drugs are administered intravenously within a short period during an anesthetic, it can be difficult to determine the exact cause of the reaction. An allergist may have to perform specific allergy testing after the recovery period.

In France, patients who develop reactions to medications administered for anesthesia are generally referred to a regional, government-run allergy center. At these centers, allergists have determined that the most likely agents to cause significant allergic reactions in anesthesia are those that are used to relax muscles. The administration of antibiotics and exposure to latex are also common causes. The latter two substances are obviously not anesthetics, but they nevertheless come into contact with the body during surgery. Latex allergy has become alarmingly common, especially among health care workers and patients who require frequent medical procedures, and has led to major changes in the manufacture of surgical implements and other health care equipment. Even though allergic responses to medications during surgery may be severe, early recognition and administration of appropriate therapies can result in complete resolution of symptoms and signs of the attack.

One of the most severe reactions to anesthetic medications is much rarer than the allergies mentioned above. Patients who develop *malignant hyperthermia* have a genetic muscle disorder in which they function quite normally in life unless they are exposed to a few types of anesthetic medications. The condition is usually unsuspected because it has no manifestations in normal daily living and therefore tends to occur unexpectedly during or soon after an anesthetic is administered. Wild changes in heart rate, blood pressure, and ventilation parameters are accompanied eventually by a severely elevated temperature and, often, severe muscle rigidity. These changes can cause injury to various different organs or even lead to death. To make matters more complicated, many patients who have malignant hyperthermia can undergo anesthesia without a reaction—even multiple times—before they eventually develop signs of this problem during or after an anesthetic. A genetic mutation is responsible for susceptibility to malignant hyperthermia, and this disorder occurs in about 1 of 5,000 to 60,000 anesthetic cases in adults, depending on geography. Because the mutation may be inherited, a family history of any suspicious event during anesthesia is an important clue to the anesthesiologist. Given its rarity, it is entirely possible for an anesthesiologist to work his or her entire career without ever encountering a case of malignant hyperthermia. Fortunately, as with allergic reactions, early recognition and therapy usually provide a good outcome for patients with this condition.

Several specific body parts or organ systems may be damaged during the process of administering anesthesia. These injuries may result from the medications themselves, the equipment, or the efforts of the provider. Eye injuries, especially external scratches called *corneal abrasions*, are not rare but have mysterious causes. The provider may inadvertently rub against the unprotected eye while looking into the airway or performing some other procedure, or patients may rub their own eyes as they awaken. These abrasions are not serious but are quite uncomfortable. They generally heal within 24 hours.

More severe cases of visual compromise or complete blindness may occur when patients are under general anesthesia. These injuries can happen in patients having operations in the prone (face-down) position, especially if the surgery is of prolonged duration. This position may result in an elevation of pressure inside the eye at a time when overall blood flow to the tissues may be compromised by anesthetic effects or by blood loss. Blood flow to the retina, where the actual cells of vision are found, is reduced, and cellular injury or cell death can ensue, resulting in visual compromise that is sometimes permanent. Surgical procedures that result in a large amount of blood loss or low blood pressure likewise predispose patients to these injuries.

Another risk factor for visual impairment in patients under anesthesia is the use of cardiopulmonary bypass during heart operations. Reports of the overall incidence of visual loss during anesthesia vary widely, from 0.002 percent to 0.2 percent of all cases. Like many adverse outcomes in medicine, this problem is probably related to multiple factors, and continued research is necessary to discern the exact causes and best means of preventing the problem. As recognition of visual loss during anesthesia has grown, so has vigilance for risk factors that can be altered.

Although most visual loss in anesthesia occurs indirectly as a result of blood flow alterations, injuries to the mouth, throat, and airway are generally due to direct physical trauma. Broken or lost teeth are among the most common complications in anesthesia and are a result of airway manipulation that is necessary for placement of the breathing tube. It is fairly common to experience a sore throat after anesthesia because of the pressure exerted on delicate tissues by the breathing tube or mask placed in your throat. However, as practitioners place these tubes into the airway, it is possible to cause injuries to the structures in this region. Lacerations and abrasions may result, but these generally heal quickly. It is also possible to cause more significant trauma to the larynx (voice box) or vocal cords during anesthesia. These injuries range from cartilage dislocation to nerve injury with vocal cord paralysis and may result in prolonged hoarseness or trouble speaking or swallowing. Such injuries require evaluation by an ear, nose, and throat physician. Some will heal spontaneously. Even when airway tubes are placed appropriately, with no apparent trauma, changes in the position of the head or neck during the surgery, or continued pressure by the inflated cuffs that are used to seal off the airway, may produce injury to a nerve in the larynx.

Injuries to the airway are most common when the nurse anesthetist or anesthesiologist encounters difficulty placing a breathing tube. This phenomenon is aptly termed *the difficult airway*, and enormous amounts of attention are paid to it in the field of anesthesiology, as well as in other fields that must provide airway management, such as emergency medicine and critical care medicine. Airways used during surgery, or in other circumstances, are usually placed after anesthesia is administered, which makes the procedure much more tolerable for patients. Unconsciousness rendered by these drugs typically leads to a cessation of breathing, however, and the immediate provision of oxygen and ventilation is imperative. Since 1993, the American Society of Anesthesiologists has sponsored guidelines to help practitioners with decision making when encountering a difficult airway. If troublesome airway management is predicted during the routine preoperative examination of the patient, the guidelines recommend that the airway tube be placed before the patient is rendered unconscious by anesthesia. This conscious airway placement is usually performed with the patient under a degree of sedation, along with topical numbing of his or her mouth and throat, so that insertion of the tube is minimally irritating.

The most concerning problems in airway management occur when anesthesiologists do not find impediments or obstacles to tube placement during the preoperative physical examination, but then have difficulty visualizing the larynx after the patients become unconscious from administration of anesthetic medications. This difficulty with visualization is usually due to the patient's anatomy. There are significant variations in how well the physical examination predicts such an inability to visualize the airway. In addition, various types of unsuspected abnormalities, such as tumors or abscesses, may obstruct the view of the vocal cords and make tube placement challenging. The difficult airway can be a mild challenge, necessitating only a change of equipment or patient position to place the tube, or it can be a true life threat, requiring the use of emergency ventilation devices or even an immediate incision in the neck to place a tracheostomy tube so that ventilation and oxygenation can be quickly resumed.

The American Society of Anesthesiologists guidelines have led to significant improvement in decision making for airway management. These recommendations allow your anesthesiologist to be more confident in assuring your safety during induction of anesthesia. In conjunction with improved training, more sophisticated tools for managing the airway, and better monitoring techniques, these guidelines appear to have resulted in a meaningful reduction in patient injury and mortality as a result of misplaced breathing tubes.

One of the most alarming complications of airway management is placement of the breathing tube into the esophagus rather than the airway. The esophagus is a long muscular tube that reaches from the back of the throat to the stomach and carries food and fluid down to the gastrointestinal tract. Anatomically, it lies just behind the larynx and can be mistaken for it under some circumstances. Placement of the tube into the esophagus usually occurs when providers have difficulty visualizing the airway, at which time the tube may be placed into the presumed correct position, without visual confirmation. Various tools are available to assist with this process, but in urgent circumstances, it may be essential to insert the tube immediately. When tracheal tube use became common in the mid-twentieth century, tube misplacement in the esophagus was not rare and resulted in a significant number of very poor outcomes. Thankfully, such tragic occurrences are much less common today, as more advanced monitors allow the anesthesiologist to confirm at once if the tube was placed in the airway and if successful ventilation is being conducted.

Nevertheless, injuries related to airway management may still occur. Inability to place a tube in the airway, despite multiple attempts and operators, occurs in roughly 1 to 2 patients out of 1,000. Anesthesiologists typically manage these situations by giving patients oxygen with a face mask and then by using other airway management tools, such as a fiberoptic bronchoscope, to guide the tube into the airway. The situation becomes critical if neither tube placement nor face mask ventilation is possible in the unconscious patient. Older analyses cite an incidence of such situations ranging from 1 to 3 patients out of 10,000. In our current health care climate, with better tools, monitoring, and awareness of this problem, there is reason to believe that this incidence will decrease.

Another complication of anesthesia related to the airway is the unexpected regurgitation of acidic stomach contents with resultant spillage into the airway. Called *pulmonary aspiration*, this was once a far too common complication of anesthesia, particularly in pregnant women. Anyone who has a stomach that is slow to empty (as in pregnancy or advanced diabetes) or a full stomach presents an increased risk of pulmonary aspiration. The damage caused by stomach contents in the airway ranges from minor wheezing and cough to severe pneumonia that requires intensive care and prolonged mechanical ventilation. Fortunately, strict observance of fasting guidelines and an increased awareness of this complication have resulted in a marked reduction in its occurrence. Pulmonary aspiration is the primary reason that anesthesiologists insist on patients avoiding food for at least six hours before surgery.

Although cardiac arrest and cardiac-related death are rare in anesthesia practice, general anesthesia commonly causes significant fluctuations in your blood pressure. Most anesthetics dilate the blood vessels, and the result is a reduction in pressure. This can be crucial because the pressure in the veins drives blood back to the heart, and if this pressure drops with the dilation of the blood vessels, so does the volume of blood that fills the heart chambers. The amount of blood pumped out with each heartbeat will fall as well, further contributing to the falling blood pressure. In addition, many anesthetic agents also reduce the strength of the pumping action by the heart, again adversely affecting blood pressure. Fortunately, most patients tolerate these declines in blood pressure quite well, and there is little or no evidence that modest declines in blood pressure correlate with adverse outcomes. If the decline in blood pressure is too severe, physicians will do what is necessary to raise it to a more acceptable level, with medications that stimulate vascular constriction or an increase in the pumping action of the heart, or with additional intravenous fluids. Most often, a combination of these modalities will be used.

Some patients are at particular risk from these falls in blood pressure. Specifically, patients who have tight or clogged vessels from atherosclerosis require higher pressures to get blood past the obstructions and into the tissue beds of crucial organs, such as the heart, brain, and kidneys. When blood flow suffers due to the fall in pressure, or due to other factors such as uncontrolled blood loss or inadequate heart pumping, cells in these critical tissues may be injured or die. The result may be stroke, heart attack, kidney failure, or generalized organ failure, and patients with these conditions have very high mortality rates. Immediate cardiac arrest from failure of blood supply to the heart itself may also occur in this setting. Such severe occurrences are fortunately uncommon, with a reported incidence of 1 in 15,000 cases. Blood pressure abnormalities *are* common, however, especially in the frail and elderly. Therefore, certain anesthetic techniques and medications are used to prevent these abnormalities from becoming too extreme.

One of the most debated complications of general anesthesia is its impact on brain function in the postoperative period. Some studies indicate prolonged cognitive dysfunction after general anesthesia, particularly in the elderly or the very young. In addition, deeper levels of anesthesia seem to predispose patients to worse brain function after surgery, which has led to a push for routine use of brain wave monitors during anesthesia. These monitors may permit guidance of anesthesia to a level that is sufficient to ensure that patients are unconscious but not excessively "deep." However, it is difficult to separate the impact of general anesthesia on cognitive postoperative brain function from the many other adverse influences on mental well-being. These include the effects of hospitalization itself, the many drugs patients receive in this period, the significant levels of postoperative pain and the medications used to treat it, changes in vital signs that occur in the perioperative period, the unfamiliar surroundings, and tissue trauma related to the surgery. Nevertheless, there is evidence that general anesthesia in very old and very young patients may have an adverse influence on brain development and function.

You may feel uneasy after reading through this long list of potential complications of general anesthesia. Most anesthesiologists do not exhaustively discuss all of these before embarking on an anesthetic plan with a patient because it would be overly intimidating and time consuming. You should feel reassured that modern anesthesia is indeed very safe based on the actual incidence of these complications, and considerably more so than it was just a couple of decades ago.

Because anesthesia was once very risky—crude instruments and unforgiving anesthetic drugs posed a true threat to life and limb—you may have come to regard anesthesia as the primary danger in the perioperative period. In fact, many of the deaths that occur in the immediate postoperative period are attributable to surgical complications, such as bleeding, failed coronary artery bypass grafts, leaking vessel repairs, or infections. It is difficult for researchers to tease out the incidence of perioperative deaths or complications caused by surgery versus those caused by the anesthetic. Such studies are few in number and tend to vary in their conclusions, depending on the source. Furthermore, surgery is divisible into many specialties and subspecialties. Surgeons tend to examine and report mishaps and adverse events within their individual practice areas, not throughout the entire spectrum of surgical treatment. In anesthesiology, there is a tendency to group many surgical types together and analyze adverse outcomes. Exceptions do exist, and detailed information is certainly available on certain subtypes of anesthesia, such as obstetric anesthesia, cardiac anesthesia, and pediatric anesthesia.

Thus, the means of collecting and analyzing information about complications attributable to anesthesia are quite variable. Large databases of acute complications in the postoperative period, amassed and analyzed by anesthesiologists, suggest that most life-threatening complications are not directly attributable to anesthesia. Surgical trauma, although not perceived by the anesthetized patient, is a significant injury to the body. Depending on the site and magnitude of tissue trauma from surgery, many adverse physiological responses may be set into motion by incision, dissection, and tissue removal. These responses include the release of inflammatory chemicals (which are valuable at the site of surgery but not as they spread throughout the body), a propensity for clotting to occur throughout the body, the release of cellular elements into the bloodstream, activation of reflex systems that liberate stress hormones, and the many maladaptive physiological effects that these responses have on the various organ systems.

The far-reaching impact of these damaging response chemicals may include stroke, heart attack, kidney failure, and an infectionlike state called *systemic inflammatory response syndrome*. The latter often leads to shock, failure of multiple organ systems, and high mortality rates. Obviously, none of these things will occur in the vast majority of surgical patients. However, risks are accentuated in patients with pre-existing illnesses and with increasing magnitude and duration of surgery. Up to 5 percent of patients who survive hospitalization for major surgery without apparent problems will later succumb to natural processes or complications of the procedure in the subsequent year. Although such deaths are obviously not directly attributable to anesthetic interventions, research is ongoing to determine whether techniques in anesthesia may have longer-term consequences than previously understood.

Some calamities, such as failure to provide adequate oxygenation and ventilation, are clearly attributable only to anesthesia management, and others, such as severe hemorrhage, are due to surgical manipulations. Many complications, however, may be regarded as shared between the two specialties because the patient is managed by both practitioners. The surgical and anesthetic process involves many components. These include, from the anesthesia side, placing intravenous catheters, diluting the blood with fluids, injecting potent medications that cause unconsciousness, placing airway devices, ventilating the lungs with a variety of gas mixtures, manipulating the central nervous system and the cardiovascular system with pharmacological agents, estimating fluid and blood losses and providing replacements, manipulating body temperature, and dulling pain receptors with drugs or local anesthetics. Surgical interventions entail cutting through the skin and other tissues, cauterizing bleeding sites, bluntly traumatizing tissues with instruments and retractors, removing and repairing organs or tissues, placing stents or drains, and suturing multiple layers of tissue. Together, these components must be seen as necessary manipulations that can have profound impact on your normal physiology.

It is important to realize that the time spent in the operating room and during the first several days after surgery are part of one prolonged perioperative period. Getting through the operation is only part of the challenge. Most perioperative heart attacks, deaths, organ failures, and strokes occur not in the operating room or in the recovery room, but in the first few days after the operation. Indeed, death in the operating room is very rare because the patient is attended by constant monitoring of vital respiratory, neurological, and cardiovascular parameters, and therapy is closely adjusted to address any evident changes in the patient's physiology on a second-to-second basis. The perioperative period of the average major surgery includes the time spent in the operating room plus the next 72 to 96 hours of initial healing and resumption of normal physiological processes. But only 2 to 5 percent of this crucial perioperative period is actually spent in the operating room. The patient spends the remaining portion in a hospital room or intensive care unit bed. In patient care units, nurses are responsible for several or even dozens of patients. The ratio of caregivers, and the availability of diagnostic and management tools at their disposal, are far less optimal than in the operating room. This is unavoidable because the health care system does not have the financial resources or staffing to keep patients in an operating room–like setting for 96 hours, awaiting the return of normal physiology.

Many complications, then, are a function of the *entire perioperative process*. They are not attributable solely to either surgery or anesthesia but are an inescapable consequence of the abnormal conditions that exist during an operation and the immediate postsurgical phase. These conditions are imposed on your body by both surgery and anesthesia, and often converge with your underlying medical problems. Anesthesiologists appreciate the importance of surgical therapy to correct a particular disease state, and by participating in the process, they predictably contribute to the potential for organ injury.

If 1 million patients volunteered for general anesthesia of a certain duration but did not undergo surgery, and we compared their postoperative course to 1 million patients who underwent the same duration of anesthesia while an invasive surgical process was undertaken, I have no doubt that the first group would have far fewer complications or deaths than the second (this study has not been performed). After such a study, we could triumphantly proclaim the safety and innocuousness of anesthesia. But we do not anesthetize patients to give them a good rest; we do it to facilitate what the surgeon must do to treat them. Therefore, anesthesia and surgery are bound together in a complex interaction, the focus of which is to see you, the patient, safely through the operative experience. And while the two specialties do occasionally find themselves in conflict over various matters—from timeliness, to monitoring techniques, to the therapies that must be provided in the operating room—it is a tribute to both professions that most patients do so well.

Many of the adverse outcomes that I have referred to as shared are unavoidable results of necessary tissue trauma during surgery. In recent years, anesthesiologists have begun to focus on ways of reducing these ill effects of the perioperative process. By numbing affected areas of the body with local anesthetic agents before the end of surgery, the degree of the surgical stress response can be reduced, and many postoperative complications can be reduced or avoided. Whether this is done by injecting local anesthetics in your incision as the wound is closed or by some type of regional anesthetic placed by your anesthesiologist before surgery, there are measurable, salutary effects. Pain control is the most obvious one, but other aspects of the postoperative stress response are also affected. This can improve your satisfaction and rehabilitation and even favorably affect overall perioperative complications and mortality. It is the nature and impact of regional anesthetic techniques with which the remainder of this book is concerned.

Chapter 5
Regional Anesthesia

 Why is it called *regional* anesthesia?

How do local anesthetics work?

What are the different types of regional anesthesia?

Will I be in less pain after surgery with regional anesthesia than with medications alone?

What is the difference between regional anesthesia and general anesthesia?

Can regional and general anesthesia complement one another?

How will my outcome be different after regional and general anesthesia?

The major categories of anesthesia—general and regional—were developed in parallel in the late nineteenth century and throughout the twentieth century. Regional anesthesia involves the *numbing* of a part of your body, rendering it incapable of sensation. This has many theoretical benefits, including the obvious one: during the operation, and for a variable period thereafter, your body senses little or no pain (table 5.1). Regional anesthesia can be employed to provide this pain relief for the duration of the surgery only, or it can be used to control pain for hours to days afterward. Either way, most nerve blocks are placed before the operation to take full advantage of the pain relief provided (figure 5.1).

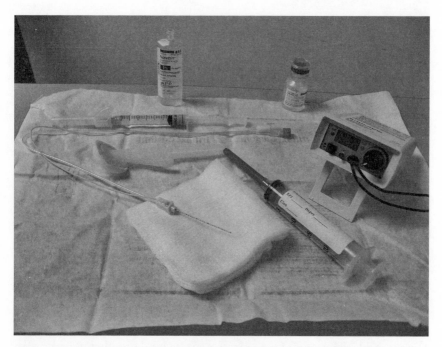

Figure 5.1 Nerve blocks may be placed in the operating room or in a preoperative holding area. Although blocks that set up rapidly, such as a spinal anesthetic, are usually placed in the operating room, those that require more time to gain access to the nerves, and therefore set up more slowly, are ideally done in a holding area well before the operation is scheduled. This approach avoids the time and space constraints of the operating room, while still permitting sedation, oxygen administration, monitoring, and ongoing observation of the patient. Shown are the tools necessary for a typical peripheral nerve block, including a prep-stick for skin sterilization, the nerve stimulator, stimulating needle, and local anesthetic solutions.

Regional anesthetic techniques require the injection of local anesthetic drugs, which are related to the procaine (Novocain) that you may be familiar with from the dentist's office. These medications interrupt nerve conduction at either the spinal nerve root level, in the case of spinal and epidural nerve blocks, or further out in the nervous system, in the peripheral nerves. The peripheral nerves stretch from the central portion of the nervous system, the brain and spinal cord, to the various destinations throughout the body to which they provide innervation. These peripheral nerves contain a mixture of nerve fibers that provide sensation to different

Table 5.1 Characteristics of regional anesthesia

Unable to move affected muscles

Unable to sense pain in affected region

Unable to sense position or temperature in affected region

Extremity may feel as if it's "floating in space"

Warmth and blood vessel dilation of affected region

parts of the body and provide movement (or *motor*) impulses to the muscles in the same areas.

Local anesthetics placed in the spine are categorized as *neuraxial* regional anesthesia techniques. Injection of local anesthetics into the vicinity of nerves after they have left the spinal cord and its protective elements, and are en route to the various tissues of your body, are termed *peripheral nerve* regional techniques (table 5.2). The impact on nerve function is the same in both types of regional anesthesia: the local anesthetic medication stops nerves from conducting impulses. Technically, these agents bind to and inactivate sodium ion channels that permit the flow of electric current along a nerve. Hence, there is an interruption, or *block*, of nerve communication. This means that sensation from the part of your body affected by the nerve block can no longer enter the central portion of the nervous system. Pain or other sensations can no longer be perceived by that part of the body. You may describe this as *numbness*, but to the anesthesiologist, this is *anesthesia* of the blocked part of the body. In addition, the affected portion of your body cannot respond to motor nerve impulses sent from the brain and spinal cord to the muscle tissue beyond the block, and therefore, the muscles of that body part temporarily relax. Muscles of the regions that are effectively anesthetized with regional anesthesia cannot be directed to move. This is most obvious if you receive a nerve block to an arm or leg.

Regional anesthesia provides a high quality of pain relief after surgeries that usually produce significant discomfort in patients. In studies evaluating different surgeries and settings, regional anesthesia techniques have produced better pain relief in the postoperative period than the use of opioid drugs, such as morphine. This improved pain relief ranges from a few hours (or even a full day) for a single-injection peripheral nerve block to several days for ongoing infusions of local anesthetics into *nerve block*

Table 5.2 **Types of nerve blocks**

1. Neuraxial blocks (involves the spine): Single or continuous
   Spinal
   Epidural
   Caudal (seldom used in adults)

2. Peripheral nerve blocks (outside the spine): Single or continuous
   Trunk (chest, abdomen, back)
   Upper extremity
   Lower extremity

catheters. To administer these catheter techniques, also referred to as *continuous* blocks, providers insert a very small, flexible tube, or *catheter*, into the patient during the nerve block procedure to continually carry local anesthetic solution from a small bedside pump to the appropriate nerve area. The catheters are placed at the site of the block—either in the spine, for an epidural-type block, or in the arm, leg, or trunk, for a peripheral nerve–type block. The catheter provides an ongoing block of sensation to the affected area of your body. The advantages of nerve blocks have been demonstrated not only by patient reports of reduced pain scores, but also by the reduction in pain medication required beyond the relief provided by the local anesthetics. Most patients who receive regional anesthetics consume significantly less pain medication and report a higher quality of pain relief after surgery.

Besides controlling pain, regional anesthesia has a number of important benefits (table 5.3). To understand them, you must consider how your body actually senses unpleasant conditions. A painful stimulus anywhere in your body is detected by sensory nerve endings and transferred back to the spinal cord, where the message is modified and sent to the brain. Pain is then perceived, or brought into your consciousness, and an action, such as moving away from the painful stimulus, is initiated. However, your spinal cord plays more than just the role of relaying messages to the brain. The spinal cord often acts as one part of a simple reflex arc and directs the injured part of your body to move away from the source of damage immediately, before your brain has even sensed what has happened. This reflex has obvious survival advantages—allowing your hand to remain on the hot stove while processing the incoming sensory information and for-

Table 5.3 **Benefits of regional anesthesia**

Provides superior pain control

Reduces postoperative nausea (by sparing injection of opioid drugs)

May reduce chronic incisional pain after surgery

Blocks the stress response to surgical trauma (inflammation)

Allows some options with degree of sedation in operating room

Avoids airway manipulation (in some cases; depends on type of block)

Is favorable for patients with sleep apnea

Allows earlier recovery of bowel function

May reduce mortality

May reduce blood clots after surgery

May reduce heart attack after surgery

May reduce respiratory failure after surgery

Allows earlier participation in rehabilitation and physical therapy

Allows earlier hospital discharge after major joint replacements

---

mulating a response would be disastrous. From this painful experience, the brain *learns* that this activity should not be repeated, while your spinal cord reflexively minimizes damage to the injured part by pulling it away as quickly as possible.

Your spinal cord plays another important role in the processing of painful stimuli, albeit one that may be detrimental. Incoming messages of pain or injury, often referred to as *noxious* stimuli, may lead to a self-amplifying excitation of nerve cells in certain areas of the cord, termed the *wind-up phenomenon*. This can actually lead to an intensification of the pain sensed, even after the injury itself has abated. In this disordered response, certain nerve cells in the spinal cord that receive and process pain impulses actively increase their excitability, creating a sort of reverberating circuit of painful impulses that can take on a life of its own. Under these circumstances, the pain that an individual perceives actually begins to outgrow the pain stimulus itself, both in magnitude and duration. It can become, in certain cases, self-perpetuating, resulting in a chronic pain state even after the damaging stimulus is long gone.

Because pain stimuli are blocked from reaching your spinal cord when providers administer regional anesthesia, this spinal cord wind-up phenomenon can be avoided entirely, or at least reduced. In fact, many chronic pain syndromes, once established, are managed with nerve blockade to interrupt or control the abnormal pain process. This use of nerve blocks is well-established in many of these chronic pain situations, though such treatment is not always the right answer and sometimes provides only temporary relief. Experimental evidence in animals suggests that preventing the spinal cord from receiving painful impulses even before a traumatic episode (such as surgery) occurs is useful to reduce the overall pain burden, even when the nerve block has completely worn off. This concept is termed *pre-emptive analgesia* because the pain is prevented before it occurs. However, pre-emptive analgesia has been difficult to study in patients, and its benefits have not been consistently borne out in clinical trials. Lately, pain researchers have been focused on the phenomenon of *chronic postsurgical pain*. Many patients who undergo certain types of surgery, such as lung or breast surgery, develop ongoing, unrelenting pain in the area of the incision. Regional anesthesia blocks used for postoperative pain control in these and other types of surgery may reduce the frequency and severity of postsurgical pain. Research is ongoing to fully elucidate the benefits of regional blocks in this setting.

Regional anesthesia also affects the stress response your body develops after surgery. When you experience pain after surgery, your body mounts both a *peripheral* (at the site of injury) and a *central* (in the central nervous system) stress response. The peripheral response involves the release of local inflammatory molecules in the surgical area, some of which may initiate adverse or undesirable effects when they are carried throughout your body. Physicians can block this process, at least in part, by injecting local anesthetics in the surgical region or by administering anti-inflammatory medications. The central stress response to surgical trauma is more severe than the peripheral response. During a central response, nerve messages related to tissue injury are carried to your central nervous system (the brain and spinal cord), which mediates a systemic reaction that includes the release of potent hormones and results in changes in your pulse, blood pressure, metabolism, and blood-clotting mechanism. Many of these changes, when unchecked, are potentially harmful to your body. Regional anesthesia, unlike general anesthesia, can effectively block the central stress responses and help to avert this bodily self-injury. This important benefit is secondary both to the pain relief that you experience from regional anesthesia (since pain is a stress in and of itself) and to the control of neurological and biochemical stress mechanisms of which you are unaware.

When a regional technique is used, some patients prefer to remain relatively lightly sedated during the procedure because they may fear the loss of control associated with deep unconsciousness. Some even wish to watch the progress of their surgery, for example, by observing the video monitor during a knee arthroscopy. You should discuss this possibility with your surgeon before the operation because many surgeons prefer to avoid the distraction of conversation with a patient while operating. Most patients, in my experience, will elect to receive a regional anesthetic, whether it is a spinal, an epidural, or a peripheral nerve block, in combination with a greater degree of sedation so that they are unconscious (with intravenous medications) and are unaware of the goings-on in the operating room.

When asked whether they would prefer regional or general anesthesia, most patients will reply, "Just put me out," or, "I don't want to know anything in the operating room, so give me a general anesthetic." It is not essential for you to undergo general anesthesia to be unaware of events in the operating room—an effective nerve block with sedation can provide the same result—and the desire to be unconscious should not determine your preference for a certain type of anesthesia. Anesthesiologists commonly provide sedation and a light plane of unconsciousness along with a regional anesthetic block, with a high degree of patient satisfaction.

General anesthesia is in essence a pharmacological coma, necessitating some type of airway and breathing support in most patients. In contrast, when your surgical site is anesthetized effectively with a regional anesthetic and is profoundly numb, only modest amounts of sedation are required for you to sleep throughout the procedure. This type of anesthesia allows you to be unconscious and unaware of events in the operating room, yet enables you to maintain enough muscle tone and strength to breathe on your own. Drugs used for sedation are generally very pleasant and can make the surgical experience quite tolerable. Overall, patients experience fewer side effects after undergoing regional anesthesia compared with general anesthesia for the same procedure.

Being able to breathe on your own during surgery can be an important benefit of regional anesthesia. Certain individuals have physical attributes that make it difficult for a provider to place a breathing tube, and others have had difficulty with breathing tubes during past experiences with anesthesia. Such situations can be life threatening if not handled appropriately. If general anesthesia is necessary for surgeries in patients with difficult airways, the anesthesiologist will usually place the breathing tube while the patient is awake, before the induction of general anesthesia. This procedure requires the anesthesiologist to numb the patient's mouth and throat, use a bronchoscope or other visualizing device to see the airway, and then insert the breathing tube with the scope. When capably done, patients tolerate this procedure fairly well, but few would ever elect to undergo it if a choice were available. For patients with difficult airways, regional anesthesia with light sedation is ideal if the nature of the surgery allows its use. However, anesthesiologists must be certain of the effectiveness of a regional block for surgery and be prepared to intubate the awake patient's airway on short notice in the operating room if the regional anesthetic becomes inadequate for some reason (for example, if the surgical duration is prolonged and a spinal block begins to wear off).

An increasing number of patients in the United States are at risk for obstructive sleep apnea, largely due to high obesity rates. Patients who have sleep apnea are more likely to have difficult-to-manage airways and have trouble recovering from medications typically used for general anesthesia, especially opioid pain medications. The opioid drugs depress respirations and are an almost universal component of general anesthesia. Regional anesthesia with very light sedation (to avoid respiratory depression and obstruction of the airway) is an ideal anesthetic technique for surgical patients with sleep apnea. Long-lasting or continuous nerve block techniques reduce the consumption of opioid medications in the postoperative period, which further enhances patient safety in this setting. This is further discussed in chapter 9.

Regional anesthesia interrupts your body's normal coagulation response to surgery. Particularly in orthopedic surgery, patients tend to develop blood clots as a result of the body's exuberant attempts to stop surgical bleeding. Clotting is life sparing, but only in the region in which you have been injured. Elsewhere, it becomes injurious, or even life threatening. Various regional anesthesia techniques, particularly spinal and epidural anesthesia, seem to reduce postoperative blood clots. As a result, there is a lower threat of clots breaking loose, circulating, and potentially compromising your heart and lung function, a phenomenon known as *pulmonary embolism*. These clots are some of the most dreaded complications of surgery. Because blood flow to the lower extremities is increased by regional anesthesia, there is less of a tendency for these clots to occur. However, as orthopedic surgeons have become more adamant about prescribing postoperative anti-clotting medications, the benefits of regional anesthesia techniques in this area have become less prominent.

An additional benefit of regional anesthesia relates to surgical blood loss: because dilated blood vessels tend to have lower pressures inside them, regional anesthetic techniques reduce bleeding in the operating room and reduce the requirement for blood transfusions. This outcome has been best established in orthopedic patients undergoing lower extremity surgeries involving their hips and knees, under spinal or epidural anesthesia.

Regional anesthesia can also help you recover your bowel function earlier after surgery. After many procedures, especially those in the abdomen, patients may develop a condition called *ileus,* which involves a lack of motility of the intestine and difficulty with digestion. Ileus may in turn slow a patient's recovery, as ingestion of nutrients and elimination are delayed. It is an inconvenience at the very least, and can have a truly detrimental impact on the recovery process. Epidural anesthesia, when maintained for pain control for several days after abdominal operations, reduces the development of ileus and allows gastric suction tubes to be removed earlier, with quicker resumption of eating and, in some cases, an earlier discharge from the hospital. When the primary means of controlling postoperative pain is with morphine or similar drugs given by injection or with a patient-controlled analgesia (PCA) apparatus, such as a morphine pump, at the bedside, these advantages are lost.

When your pain is controlled in the operating room and in the postoperative period, your central response to pain is reduced or prevented. Because the stress response to pain has adverse effects on various organ systems in your body, preventing it is likely to be beneficial, resulting in shorter hospital stays and lower mortality. Although physicians have documented reductions in inflammation and mediators of the stress response in patients who underwent surgery with regional anesthesia, the overall impact of this approach on identifiable patient outcomes is not yet known.

Anesthesiologists are divided about the idea that regional anesthesia can reduce the most feared complications of major surgeries, such as heart attack and cardiac death. Many practitioners of regional anesthesia firmly believe that regional techniques are likely to improve outcomes in patients with significant heart or vascular disease. Few studies confirm this assertion, however, and the studies that do exist have shown no significant, consistent difference in outcome between patients who have undergone general anesthesia and those who have had regional anesthesia. Proponents of regional anesthesia argue that virtually all of these studies have been too small to detect any but very large differences in outcome between the groups. For example, if regional anesthesia, or any type of medical intervention, were to decrease the rate of heart attacks in a group of patients from 3 percent to 2 percent (a notable one-third reduction), you would likely recognize this as an important benefit, especially when thousands of patients are considered. The problem is that many of the anesthesia trials have included only twenty to fifty patients in each group, and the detection of such a change (from a 3 percent to a 2 percent occurrence) is difficult with such low numbers. Statistically, much larger groups would be required for meaningful comparison.

One of the ways to compensate for small numbers of patients in multiple trials is to combine the results of many trials together, a technique called *meta-analysis*. Researchers applied this statistical method in the analysis of some 120 small, randomized trials that had compared regional and general anesthesia techniques in more than 9,000 patients. The results appeared to favor regional techniques for several different outcomes. The authors of this study concluded that, with regional anesthesia, there was a 33 percent reduction in heart attack, a 40 percent reduction in postoperative pneumonia, and a 30 percent reduction in blood clots in the lower extremities. There was also a 25 percent reduction in pulmonary embolism. Blood loss and transfusion requirements were significantly reduced in the groups who underwent regional anesthesia. Most importantly, mortality was reduced by 33 percent when providers incorporated regional blocks into the anesthetic. These results remain controversial, however, and physicians continue to await large, prospective, randomized trials that compare outcomes from general and from regional anesthesia.

In the outpatient setting, you come to the hospital for surgery and return home on the same day. Regional anesthesia is in line with the goals in this setting: rapid awakening, minimal postoperative side effects, and early discharge and rehabilitation. If you have been rendered numb at the operative site by regional anesthesia, you need less anesthesia medication to sleep comfortably through surgery. Therefore, integration of regional anesthesia into your anesthetic plan, whether it is the primary mode of anesthesia or an addition to a general anesthetic, allows for the use of less systemic anesthetic drugs, a more rapid emergence from anesthesia, and better pain control on arrival in the post-anesthesia care unit (PACU).

In many cases, when regional blocks are a prominent part of the anesthetic plan, patients come to consciousness quickly enough to bypass the PACU altogether, returning to the outpatient nursing unit to begin preparing for discharge home. This increases patient and family satisfaction.

For people who must undergo a major inpatient orthopedic surgery, such as total hip or knee replacement, or an outpatient procedure requiring intense rehabilitation, such as ligament repairs of the knee, nerve blocks are definitely worth consideration. Patients having such procedures do well with regional anesthesia. Several studies have shown that regional techniques, particularly continuous catheter peripheral nerve blocks, allow earlier participation in physical therapy and a greater range of pain-free extremity motion in the early postoperative period than with general anesthetics followed by opioid medications. Other types of surgery that result in significant postoperative pain that could delay recovery, and which lend themselves to the use of regional anesthetic techniques, include surgeries of the pelvis, abdomen, or chest, or the removal or manipulation of large amounts or multiple layers of tissue, such as hernia repair.

Chapter 6

Spinal Anesthesia and Epidural Anesthesia

 What is neuraxial regional anesthesia and how is it performed?

What is *spinal* anesthesia?

What is *epidural* anesthesia?

When is a spinal anesthetic useful?

How is epidural different from spinal anesthesia?

How does my anesthesiologist know where to put an epidural in my spine?

When is a continuous epidural useful?

What are the most common side effects of neuraxial regional anesthetics?

Neuraxial regional anesthesia is a process involving the injection of local anesthetics into the spine to produce spinal and epidural nerve blocks. Neuraxial regional anesthetics are common and can be used for many different surgeries in the lower body, such as surgery of the prostate, genitals, legs, anus, and any soft tissues of the waist area (such as hernia repair) (table 6.1). In addition, most non-emergency cesarean sections are performed with neuraxial regional anesthesia, which allows the mother to be awake for delivery.

There are two types of neuraxial regional anesthesia: spinal and epidural. With both types, anesthesiologists inject the local anesthetic medi-

Table 6.1   **Common surgeries involving neuraxial anesthesia**

Obstetrics (labor pain, cesarean section births)

Prostate surgery

Genital or anal surgery

Hernia surgery

Orthopedic lower extremity surgery, especially hip and knee

Abdominal, pelvic, or thoracic procedures (epidurals commonly used for postoperative pain)

cation within the spine, where it acts on the delicate nerve roots that have emerged from the spinal cord. The spinal cord has many different levels, or segments; these segments supply nerves that allow for sensation and muscle movement in different regions of the body. At each segment, multiple tiny nerve rootlets emerge from the front (muscle control fibers) and back (sensation fibers) of the cord. These rootlets then come together to form a spinal nerve root, which exits the spinal canal. The roots then acquire fibers from the sympathetic (fight or flight) nervous system, which controls many involuntary functions of the body, before proceeding to the outlying areas of the body, where they are designated as *peripheral* nerves.

There are thirty-one spinal cord levels and twenty-nine spinal vertebrae, or *backbones*, in the adult human body. In the fetus, the spinal cord levels and spinal vertebrae are at approximately the same level. However, with on-going growth and development, the spinal bones outpace the cord, which grows substantially less than the bones. As a result, by adulthood, the spinal cord ends about two-thirds of the way down the spinal canal from the brain. The nerve roots leaving the lower portion of the cord continue downward to exit the spine in the lowest part of the back (the lumbar and sacral levels). Spinal and epidural blocks work on the spinal nerve roots— the fragile, unprotected fibers that have just emerged from the cord.

Why would your anesthesiologist recommend a spinal or epidural nerve block? These types of blocks provide a comfortable, safe anesthetic for various procedures on the lower extremities and the lower trunk. Neuraxial regional anesthesia can save you the discomfort of having a breathing tube in your throat, which is usually necessary in general anesthesia. If you wish to be alert and functional as soon as possible after surgery, neuraxial anesthesia with light sedation is ideal. Any pain you may experience in the immediate postoperative period can be well controlled with this type of anesthesia, and the need for postoperative opioids is usually reduced (if not abolished entirely). If you have ever had nausea or vomiting after general anesthesia, neuraxial regional anesthesia may also reduce the chance of these side effects by as much as 50 percent.

A spinal or epidural anesthetic may sound painful or uncomfortable because the spinal canal is located deep inside your back. It is normal to feel apprehensive about these procedures. By explaining how they are performed, I hope to make them less mysterious and potentially frightening for anyone who needs them or may benefit from them.

Both epidural and spinal blocks can be performed with the patient sitting or lying on one side. After placing appropriate vital sign monitors and providing sedation, your anesthesiologist will disinfect and then numb your skin and underlying tissue with a small dose of local anesthetic. With sedation and reassurance to prepare you for the block, as well as a liberal application of local anesthetic in the skin, you will likely feel only pressure from the needle used to administer the anesthetic. Many patients are surprised at how little discomfort they experience.

To perform a spinal, or *subarachnoid*, block, the anesthesiologist inserts a long, thin needle through the patient's skin, underlying tissues, and spinal ligaments, and into the sac of fluid that protects the spinal cord (called the *subarachnoid space*). Typically, the block is done in the lower (lumbar) portion of the back, around the third or fourth lumbar interspace, because the spinal cord ends above this level and is therefore protected from the procedure (figure 6.1). After the anesthesiologist confirms the entry of the needle into the subarachnoid space by the appearance of clear fluid in the needle hub, he or she injects a small dose of local anesthetic into the space. Because the appropriate placement of the needle is confirmed by the clear cerebrospinal fluid, a spinal block is a very reliable technique. Most other types of nerve blocks do not allow such clear evidence of appropriate needle tip placement near the nerves that need to be anesthetized.

After injection of local anesthetic, your nerve roots, which do not have the protective covering of other nerves in your body, are quickly subjected to a blockade of electrical conduction. Where in your body will you lose sensation during a spinal block? The answer depends on multiple factors, including the dose of drug injected (higher doses usually achieve a higher

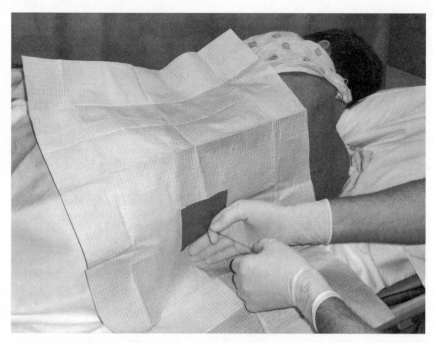

Figure 6.1 This patient is about to undergo injection of a spinal anesthetic. He has received intravenous sedation to reduce anxiety but remains awake and able to provide feedback to the anesthesiologist. The spinal block is usually placed in the lower lumbar spine, below the level at which the spinal cord ends. A very small quantity of lidocaine has been injected into the skin at the site of the spinal to make the process painless, though many patients feel some degree of pressure. Spinal blocks can be placed with the patient either sitting or lying on one side.

level block), the density of the solution, and your physical position when the drug is injected (table 6.2). Anesthesiologists can use gravity to affect specific nerve roots by having a patient lie on his or her operative side and by injecting a *hyperbaric*, or dense, local anesthetic solution. For example, an anesthesiologist might administer a hyperbaric local anesthetic solution during a spinal block for a surgical procedure on your right knee while you are lying on your right side. Because the hyperbaric solution is denser than cerebrospinal fluid, it will sink toward the right-sided nerve roots. As a result, the block will be denser and last longer on the operative (right) side than on the nonoperative side. Many patients receiving this type of one-sided spinal block are able to move their nonoperative leg by the time they

Table 6.2 Factors affecting the spread of a spinal block

Major factors:

Density of injected solution

Position of patient during (and immediately after) injection

Total dose of drug

Minor factors:

Patient height

Level of placement

reach the post-anesthesia care unit (PACU), even though the operative leg remains comfortable and numb.

Within several minutes of receiving a spinal nerve block, you will begin to sense its effects, and your vital signs may change. You may initially experience a warm sensation and then numbness or heaviness in the legs and up to the waist. Sometimes patients feel as if their affected body part is floating. You may not sense anything below the waist. Because of the sedation you receive before a spinal block, you will likely remember very little of this process. If you subsequently have surgery, you will probably sleep comfortably under sedation, experiencing no pain but perhaps noting an occasional sense of pulling or vibration in the lower body. According to your preferences and the severity of any underlying medical problems you may have, you may be sedated lightly, or deeply enough to make sure you have no conscious experience.

How long your spinal block lasts depends on the dose and type of anesthesia medication you are given (certain additives can also prolong the spinal block). Local anesthetic agents, such as procaine (Novocain), reliably produce blocks that last less than 60 minutes. Agents of intermediate duration, such as bupivacaine (Marcaine), last one to two hours, and some medications, such as tetracaine, last longer than two hours. After the anesthesiologist places the spinal block, however, its duration is fixed, and it cannot be prolonged unless he or she performs another block. When anesthesiologists refer to the term *duration*, they mean the length of time of *surgical anesthesia*, or the period during which a very deep numbness is essential for the surgeon to work. You should know that it may be another hour or so after the surgical anesthesia period before your legs are strong enough to move well.

Sometimes blocks of the spinal nerve roots must last for several hours to provide anesthesia during a process or procedure of uncertain length (such as labor or a prolonged surgery), or for several days to provide relief from pain after a major surgery. In these cases, an epidural block, which is usually continuous, is more appropriate than a spinal block. As with a spinal block, an epidural block numbs your spinal nerve roots. Instead of injecting the local anesthetic solution inside the subarachnoid sac of fluid, however, the anesthesiologist injects it into the region just outside the sac. The outer membrane of the sac is called the *dura mater*, and the area around it is termed the *epidural space*. Rather than inject drugs directly during the placement of the epidural, anesthesiologists prefer to insert a small, flexible tube, or *catheter*, through the needle and into the epidural space. This catheter remains in your back when the needle is removed and can be used to continuously or repeatedly inject local anesthetics into the epidural space to provide surgical anesthesia for an operation or for labor and delivery. Likewise, the catheter can be used for ongoing postoperative pain relief. The great advantage of the epidural block is the ability to use it continuously for long periods.

Placing an epidural block is much more complex and technically de-manding than placing a spinal block. As during the placement of a spinal block, you may be seated or be lying on one side, and your anesthesiologist will ask you to curl your back to help open the spaces between your ver-tebral bones. After placing appropriate monitors and providing sedation, your anesthesiologist will prepare the skin with a disinfectant and then anesthetize the skin and underlying tissue with a small dose of local anes-thetic. Then he or she will use a needle attached to a syringe to locate the epidural space. Most commonly, this is done with a *loss of resistance* tech-nique, in which the physician applies continuous pressure on the plunger of the syringe until the resistance of the major ligament of the posterior spinal canal gives way. This lets the physician know that the epidural space has been entered. The catheter is then gently inserted into the spinal canal, where it most commonly moves off to one side or the other but is still capable of anesthetizing the nerve roots of both sides of your body as the injected solution accumulates and spreads within the canal.

Immediately after inserting the catheter, the anesthesiologist will ad-minister a small *test dose* of local anesthetic solution mixed with adrenaline to ensure that the catheter is safely and correctly placed. This test dose ensures that the catheter has not been placed inside a blood vessel (in which case the adrenaline would make the patient's heart race), or inside the spinal sac itself (in which case the small dose of local anesthetic would rapidly produce leg weakness and numbness, like a spinal block). After the anesthesiologist confirms that the catheter has been correctly placed, he or she then administers the main local anesthetic solution slowly and by gradations because it represents a much larger dose than that of a spinal block. Administering such a dose into the spinal sac would cause an undesirably high level of spinal blockade with compromise of the patient's blood pressure, heart function, breathing, and perhaps even consciousness. Only a small fraction of the drug placed in the epidural space will make its way across the protective membranes of the spinal sac and into the subarachnoid space to affect the nerve roots.

The body regions affected by an epidural anesthetic do not depend on the density of the solution or the patient's body position, as they do with spinal blockade. Instead, the major determinants of epidural block level are the drug dose administered through the epidural catheter and the spinal level at which the epidural is placed. Unlike spinal blocks, epidurals do not have to be placed below the level at which your spinal cord ends, because the epidural needle is not intended to enter the protective sac in which the spinal cord is suspended. Therefore, anesthesiologists can choose to place epidural blocks at many different spinal levels. They often place epidurals at lumbar levels for procedures or processes involving the legs and genital region, at slightly higher levels for procedures involving the middle or upper abdomen, and at mid-back (or thoracic) levels (at approximately the height of the shoulder blades) for surgeries involving the rib cage or lungs (table 6.3).

In contrast to a spinal block, the duration of an epidural block is not fixed. Because anesthesiologists usually place a catheter when they perform the initial epidural block, a patient may receive dilute solutions of local anesthetic through the catheter for days after the initial procedure. Low concentrations of opioid medications (such as morphine or fentanyl) are often included with the anesthetic in these epidural infusions. If your body becomes too numb or weak, or if you have other undesirable side effects from the anesthetic, the anesthesiologist may decrease or temporarily discontinue the infusion. A pump at your bedside will administer the infusion, or you may be given the option of pressing a button to supply your own doses of anesthetic solution through the epidural catheter. This latter option is called *patient-controlled epidural analgesia* (PCEA). PCEA

Table 6.3 Differences between spinal blocks and epidural blocks

Variable	Spinal	Epidural
Location affected by anesthetic medication	spinal nerve roots	spinal nerve roots
Place drug deposited	subarachnoid space	epidural space
Set-up time	2–5 minutes	5–20 minutes
Dose of drug	small	much larger (5–10 fold)
Determinants of block spread (i.e., what levels of the body will be affected)	density position of patient dose of drug	level of injection dose of drug
Levels of placement	lumbar spine (always)	low lumbar spine low thoracic spine middle to high thoracic spine
Length of time that block is useful for postoperative pain	up to 24 hours	up to several days (with catheter)

is similar to *patient-controlled analgesia* (PCA) in that it involves the use of a pump at the bedside to provide on-demand doses of anesthetic medications in the postoperative period. However, the patient receives medication through an epidural catheter during PCEA rather than through an intravenous (IV) catheter, as with PCA.

Epidural blocks are particularly versatile and effective in obstetric anesthesia. They are often used during labor and delivery because they provide pain relief while still allowing the mother to push with her pelvic muscles when needed (at this stage, the anesthesiologist simply discontinues the local anesthetic infusion). Epidural blocks can also be used when labor does not proceed according to plan and an urgent cesarean section must be performed. In these cases, the anesthesiologist has often already placed an epidural catheter for control of labor pain and therefore needs only to inject a more concentrated local anesthetic through the catheter to provide dense anesthesia of the lower abdomen for a surgical incision.

Besides allowing the mother to be alert and active in the birth of her baby, regional anesthesia has other important advantages in the obstetric setting. The drugs usually given for general anesthesia, both intravenously and in gaseous form, may cross the placenta and cause a newborn to require immediate resuscitation and intensive support to survive. In addition, a mother's stomach often remains full long after eating during late pregnancy, leaving her vulnerable to vomiting and lung injury during the initial phases of general anesthesia. Finally, many pregnant women gain weight dramatically in the last trimester of pregnancy due to breast hypertrophy, adipose storage, and water retention. Tissue in the neck, chin, breasts, and even inside the throat may be pronounced, which may complicate an anesthesiologist's attempts to place an airway if general anesthesia is initiated. On the other hand, drugs infused through the epidural catheter during regional anesthesia have little or no effect on the fetus and provide excellent pain relief for the mother (or even dense anesthesia, if needed for a cesarean section). For all of these reasons, regional anesthesia is the preferred method for providing anesthesia during labor and delivery.

Other uses for epidural anesthesia, in addition to obstetrics, include any lower extremity procedure that is expected to cause significant postoperative pain, such as a total hip or knee replacement or a fracture repair. Anesthesiologists can insert an epidural catheter in patients solely for postoperative pain control after using a general anesthetic for the surgery. Alternatively, the catheter can be used as a *renewable* spinal block, providing profound numbness for the surgery itself and then pain control during the first days of postoperative recovery. Epidural anesthesia is ideal for lower extremity procedures to repair diseased arteries because the continued postoperative infusion of local anesthetics may reduce the likelihood of clotting in the newly repaired vessels. Researchers attribute this decreased likelihood of clotting to increased blood flow and dilation of the vessels involved in epidural anesthesia.

Surgery that involves the pelvis, abdomen, or thoracic spine usually requires general anesthesia because it is difficult for anesthesiologists to numb the deep, visceral nerves of the body that provide sensation to the internal organs, and because the patient's muscles usually must be relaxed for such a procedure to be done. Many surgeries that require general anesthesia, however, particularly upper abdominal and thoracic surgeries, are quite painful postoperatively. Epidural anesthesia is a more effective means of controlling pain with these types of surgeries than IV opioid injections or PCA pumps that provide morphine at the bedside. Including epidural anesthesia for pain control after such surgeries has been shown to improve patient recovery, decrease postoperative *ileus* (relaxation of the bowel), and improve lung function. Such advantages are particularly important for older patients with pre-existing medical problems.

As with many medical procedures, neuraxial anesthesia has potential adverse effects (table 6.4). Both epidural and spinal blocks tend to produce a fall in blood pressure, but this is readily controlled with an injection of medication as well as an increase in fluids administered through the patient's IV catheter. (General anesthesia likewise tends to produce low blood pressure, as discussed in chapter 3.)

During needle or catheter insertion for neuraxial blocks, patients may experience a sharp discomfort called a *paresthesia* that radiates to their buttocks, pelvis, or legs. This sensation is akin to the funny bone feeling that most people have experienced—a shock-like electrical sensation that runs down to the forearm and hand and is the result of trauma to the ulnar nerve behind the elbow. There are generally no long-term consequences of a single, brief paresthesia. Continued needle advancement against the nerve that produced the paresthesia, with injection of local anesthetic solution into the nerve at that site, may result in nerve injury and possible sensory loss or weakness, and anesthesiologists will avoid any such maneuver.

Most paresthesias are benign and have no consequences. Nonetheless, the possibility of a paresthesia is the main reason that regional anesthetic

Table 6.4 Potential side effects of neuraxial blocks

Reduced blood pressure (occasionally severe)

Paresthesia or pain during placement

Lowering of body temperature

Shivering (especially with spinal blocks and in obstetrics)

Spinal (postdural puncture) headache

Itching

Weak legs until block resolves (falling hazard)

procedures should be conducted while patients are alert enough to report such sensations. Gentle advancement of the needle and constant communication between patient and anesthesiologist allows spinal and epidural blocks to proceed safely, with little likelihood of nerve injury. If you undergo one of these procedures, your anesthesiologist will ask you to speak up immediately if you feel a sharp pain or an electrical sensation. He or she needs to be aware of what you experience during the block because it is an important guide to further anesthetic procedures.

Temperature regulation in patients is a challenge for anesthesiologists in both regional and general anesthesia. After receiving general anesthesia or a neuraxial anesthetic, you may find yourself shivering in the PACU. This phenomenon is partly related to vascular dilation and heat loss from the skin, but there may be some direct effect of the anesthesia on your nervous system as well. Some patients who shiver after anesthesia deny feeling cold. Pregnant women seem to have the most vigorous shivering response to epidural or spinal anesthesia and often shiver violently in the recovery room after delivery. Warming techniques such as forced-air warming with devices kept ready in the recovery room, as well as IV medications, generally help bring the shivering under control. Even without treatment, shivering eventually subsides on its own.

You have probably heard of the *spinal headache*—a dull headache that occurs a day or so after a spinal anesthetic (or any type of needle insertion at the spine, including a myelogram or a spinal tap). Spinal headaches usually affect people when they sit up after a spinal anesthetic, but then resolve when they lie down again. This condition is the result of a hole in the dural sac, which envelops and protects the spinal cord and nerve roots. As discussed earlier in this chapter, this sac is intentionally punctured with the needle during a spinal block; it may also be perforated unintentionally during placement of an epidural. Most punctures of the dural sac close spontaneously, especially with the very small needles used for spinal blocks today. However, in a few patients, these perforations do not close on their own (larger punctures produced by an epidural needle usually do *not* close of their own accord), leading to the phenomenon of *postdural puncture*, or *spinal*, headache.

Spinal headaches are much less common today than they were even two decades ago thanks to an understanding of what causes them and the availability of smaller needles for spinal anesthetics. When a person does get a spinal headache, the anesthesiologist will usually prescribe bed rest with an increase in fluids for a 24-hour period and possibly recommend that the patient have some caffeine, which seems to help. A significant proportion of headaches will resolve with this noninvasive therapy. If they persist, the next step will usually be an *epidural blood patch*. This procedure is essentially a biological Band-aid, in which the anesthesiologist places an epidural needle at approximately the same level of the original spinal or epidural block (or myelogram). He or she draws some blood from the patient's arm at the same time and then injects the blood through the needle into the epidural space to help seal off the hole in the dural sac and stop the fluid leak. Epidural blood patches are successful on the first attempt in about nine out of ten cases. If not successful, the procedure can safely be attempted again, which increases the success rate.

❊ Despite these potential adverse effects, there are many benefits of undergoing surgery with neuraxial-type regional anesthesia rather than general anesthesia. This chapter has specifically discussed neuraxial blocks—spinal and epidural—that stop nerve conduction at the level of the spinal nerve roots and are most useful for procedures or pain involving the lower extremities or trunk. In the next chapter, I examine a different type of regional block—the peripheral nerve block.

Chapter 7

Peripheral Nerve Blocks

 What is a *peripheral* nerve?

Where are peripheral nerve blocks placed?

Which placement method is best?

What will I experience when getting a peripheral nerve block?

Can peripheral blocks be combined with other types of anesthesia?

What are the advantages of peripheral blocks for surgery and pain control?

Is a peripheral nerve block sufficient for anesthesia before surgery?

How are peripheral blocks different from neuraxial blocks?

Do peripheral nerve blocks have side effects?

How long do peripheral nerve blocks last?

The two forms of regional anesthesia are neuraxial blocks, which involve the spine, and peripheral nerve blocks. *Peripheral* refers to a nerve that has left the spinal column and is moving toward the area of the body for which it provides nervous communication, or *innervation*. This chapter focuses on peripheral nerve blockade, which may be used in combination with neuraxial anesthetic techniques or with general anesthesia. In recent years, anesthesiologists have increasingly preferred peripheral nerve blockade to neuraxial techniques to provide pain relief after many major orthopedic procedures.

To perform a peripheral nerve blockade, anesthesiologists must have a thorough understanding of the anatomy of the nervous system. At each level of the spinal cord, nerve roots emerge and move away from the vertebral column toward areas of the body that they innervate. As the nerves emerge from the vertebral column, they may form a network of nerves, called a *plexus*, in which individual nerve fibers reorganize themselves into peripheral nerves. After passing through the *brachial plexus* (a network of nerves located in the neck and armpit), the peripheral nerves of the upper extremity go on to innervate the arm and the shoulder. Two plexuses organize the nerves that innervate the leg: the *lumbar plexus*, which supplies most of the hip and thigh region as well as the knee, and the *sacral plexus*, which supplies the gluteus muscles, pelvis, backs of the thighs, and most structures below the knee. Peripheral nerves that supply the head, neck, and trunk proceed directly from the vertebral column to their destinations, without passing through a plexus.

Peripheral nerves carry information, gathered from the environment by specialized receptors, to the central nervous system (*sensory nerve fibers*). They also transmit impulses from the central nervous system to the muscles of the body (*motor nerve fibers*) (figure 7.1). The ears, nose, mouth, and eyes supply detailed information about the environment to the brain via special peripheral nerves called *cranial nerves*. Sensory nerve endings in the skin and underlying tissue, in the linings of muscles and bones, and in the ligaments conduct impulses via peripheral nerves to deliver the perception of pain, touch, temperature, and vibration. Additionally, they deliver *proprioception*, which is the person's sense of where their body is located in space.

In addition to sensory and motor information, peripheral nerves also carry information related to the control of blood vessels and sweat glands (table 7.1). Most peripheral nerves carry all of this information (called *mixed* nerves), but a few carry only sensory or motor information.

Anesthesiologists can block the transmission of information by peripheral nerves by injecting local anesthetic next to the nerve at any point as it courses through the body toward the structures it innervates. Sometimes a nerve is close enough to the surface of the skin or a mucous membrane, such as in the throat, for anesthesiologists to block it by simply applying a solution of topical local anesthetics. However, the majority of peripheral nerve blocks involve using a needle to deposit the local anesthetic solution

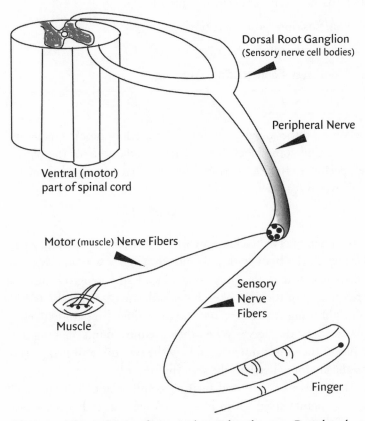

Dorsal (sensory)
part of spinal cord

Dorsal Root Ganglion
(Sensory nerve cell bodies)

Peripheral Nerve

Ventral (motor)
part of spinal cord

Motor (muscle) Nerve Fibers

Muscle

Sensory
Nerve
Fibers

Finger

Figure 7.1 The pathway of a typical peripheral nerve. Peripheral nerves carry sensation messages from the body along dedicated sensory nerve cell projections. The sensory nerve cell bodies lie in a collection near the spinal cord, *dorsal root ganglion*, at each spinal level. The same peripheral nerves also carry muscle innervation via dedicated *motor* nerve cell fibers, whose cell bodies lie within the spinal cord itself. Thus, the peripheral nerve is a collection of extremely long fibers, called *axons*, from these cell bodies near or in the spinal cord, along with supportive cells and connective tissue to ensure protection, nutrition, and an optimal milieu for electrical transmission. Within the body cavities, connections between the spinal cord and internal organs (*visceral nerves*) have a different arrangement, but these are not the direct targets of nerve blocks by anesthesiologists.

Table 7.1 Peripheral nerve functions

Skin sensation: pain, touch, temperature, vibration

Spatial sensation: position, proprioception

Motor: muscle strength, motion

Autonomics: blood vessel constriction, sweating

near the nerve. Anesthesiologists perform some nerve blocks, including most arm blocks and some blocks for the legs, at the level of the plexus. Others they perform after the peripheral nerves have emerged from the plexus, in the extremity itself.

Most peripheral nerve blockade involves inserting a needle into a particular area of the body with guidance from surface anatomy, nerve stimulation, or ultrasound imaging. Regional anesthesiologists must be intimately familiar with the path of each nerve they wish to block, its relationship to neighboring structures, and the clues they can gain by feeling the surface area above the nerve. When they use ultrasound imaging during a nerve block, they must understand how the two-dimensional picture correlates to the anatomy beneath the skin (figure 7.2).

Because the paths of nerves and their anatomic relationships are well known, the best points at which to block them have already been established; most of these points were identified in the previous century (table 7.2). New technology, such as magnetic resonance imaging and ultrasound imaging, have made it possible to describe and measure nerve positions with greater precision and have revealed a few new positions where a peripheral nerve can be blocked. Anesthesiologists usually block nerves at readily accessible points, where they can be reasonably certain the nerves are located. This procedure is very similar whether the block is guided by anatomy or by the use of ultrasound imaging (table 7.3).

Anesthesiologists may locate, or *localize*, a nerve within the body in different ways to apply local anesthetic effectively. The time-honored method, which is still in use to some degree today, is to contact the nerve with the tip of the needle, producing a *paresthesia*—an electrical buzz or brief sharp pain in the area of the nerve. This method is more effective in the

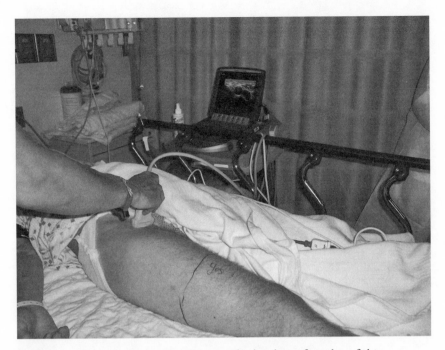

Figure 7.2 In recent years, ultrasonography has been found useful in visualizing many superficial nerves that are subject to nerve blocks for surgery and postoperative pain relief. Prior to this, anesthesiologists localized nerves by feeling anatomic landmarks at the surface of the body or extremities and using these landmarks to guide needle placement. Eventually, electrical nerve stimulation came to complement these physical landmarks and provide an enhanced degree of accuracy. Increasingly, ultrasound is being used as the primary mode of nerve localization, either alone or as a complement to electrical nerve stimulation.

upper than in the lower extremity, probably because of the more thorough sensory innervation in the arm.

With the development of peripheral nerve electrical stimulators in the 1970s, a new method of nerve localization became popular. In this technique, an anesthesiologist applies a minuscule electrical charge to a specialized needle to excite the nerve as it is approached by the tip of the needle. The excitation of the nerve results in muscle activity in the area it supplies—a rhythmic muscle *twitch*. Manipulation of the electrical current, and its impact on the strength of this twitch, allows the anesthesiologist

Table 7.2 Common sites of peripheral nerve blocks

Block name (site of block)	Area affected
Para-vertebral	Trunk (abdomen, chest wall, groin)
TAP block (abdominal wall)	Abdominal wall, groin
Rectus sheath (anterior abdomen)	Umbilical area
Brachial plexus (neck, shoulder, arm)	Entire arm
Lumbar plexus (lower back region)	Hip, front of thigh, knee
Sacral plexus (buttocks region)	Hip
Femoral nerve (upper-front thigh)	Front of thigh, knee
Sciatic nerve (upper-back thigh and buttock)	Lower leg, foot
Individual nerves of arm or leg	Hand, foot

Table 7.3 How anesthesiologists locate a nerve for blockade

Physical exam and feeling of landmark anatomy

Paresthesia (contacting the needle to nerve)

Muscle stimulation (peripheral nerve stimulation)

Through a local blood vessel (transarterial)

Ultrasound imaging

Ultrasound imaging plus muscle stimulation

to localize the needle tip to a position very close to the nerve (figure 7.3). He or she then injects the local anesthetic solution, which stops the twitch. Unlike the paresthesia method for localizing a nerve, the peripheral nerve stimulator method does not rely on eliciting an uncomfortable sensation in the patient. Paresthesias are occasionally encountered when a needle is placed for the nerve stimulator technique, and although they can still be used to aid nerve localization, the motor twitch is a preferred method of localization.

Anesthesiologists may also perform a peripheral nerve block by simply

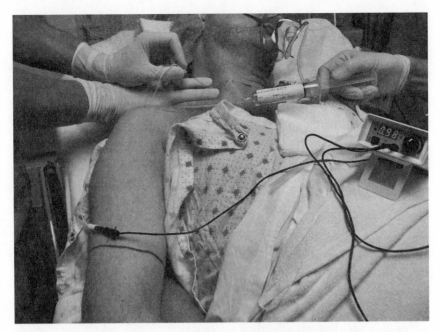

Figure 7.3 A block is placed in the lower neck to provide anesthesia for a shoulder surgery. The anesthesiologist has placed his fingers so he can feel the groove between the scalene muscles in order to guide the needle into the vicinity of the brachial plexus, which supplies nerves to the shoulder and arm. After the skin is anesthetized, a stimulating needle will be inserted into the interscalene groove until an appropriate muscle stimulation is evident in the shoulder or upper arm, indicating appropriate needle tip placement, at which time the local anesthetic will be injected. The patient is sedated but is able to provide feedback if any pain or unusual symptoms are perceived as the medication is injected.

placing the needle in the expected location of the nerve, using anatomy as a guide and without nerve stimulation or nerve contact. Usually these injections depend on physical features near the nerve, such as an arterial pulse or a bony prominence. Advocates of the nerve stimulator method believe that these types of *blind injection* are less accurate and less likely to produce an adequate block than the process of isolating individual nerves with the peripheral nerve stimulator.

✣ It is not clear that any one method of nerve localization is safer than another. However, the use of ultrasound imaging is becoming increasingly popular as a method of identifying nerves and helping guide the needle to the desired nerve. There are several advantages of using ultrasound imaging during peripheral nerve blockade. Even though nerve pathways are relatively predictable from landmarks on the body, variations in patient position and body shape may distort these landmarks. These variations introduce uncertainty in an anesthesiologist's search for nerves and may require him or her to reinsert the needle several times to localize a nerve, which increases patient discomfort. In addition, local anatomic structures located near the target nerve, such as blood vessels or the lungs, may be endangered by blind injections. Therefore, being able to *see* the anatomy beneath the skin during the block and to guide the needle accurately to the target nerve are great benefits of ultrasound imaging (figure 7.4).

Researchers have found that ultrasound guidance during a nerve block procedure reduces the number of needlesticks and needle redirections under the patient's skin, as well as the time it takes to perform the block. In addition, some (but not all) studies comparing ultrasound to other needle guidance techniques have revealed an improvement in block success rates. Because of these advantages, it is possible that ultrasound imaging will replace nerve stimulation as the preferred technique of localizing nerves in the future. On the other hand, these techniques complement each other and provide important information about both nerve anatomy and function, and therefore many anesthesiologists use them in combination.

✣ Regardless of how your anesthesiologist chooses to guide local anesthetic to your nerve, if you receive a nerve block, your experience during the procedure will likely be the same (table 7.4). As with neuraxial anesthesia, the anesthesiologist will perform the block in an operating room or in a preoperative holding area. He or she will place monitors for your heart, blood pressure, and oxygen saturation and will insert an IV in your hand or arm. In most cases, the anesthesiologist will then administer sedation medication. Because your perception and ability to communicate with the physician are important to maintain nerve block safety, the sedation will be administered in small doses to relieve anxiety and control pain but not to cause you to lose consciousness. You will remain alert enough to relate whether you feel pain in the innervated area of the body during insertion of the needle and the injection of local anesthetic solution. Such

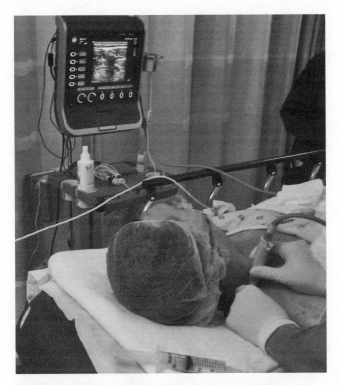

Figure 7.4 An ultrasound-guided nerve block for shoulder surgery is in progress. The ultrasound transducer probe is placed over the interscalene groove (much as the fingers were used as a guide in the nerve stimulator block in figure 7.3) to image the muscles and the nerves that lie between them. Once again, the skin is anesthetized, and a needle is placed through the numb area, to reach the vicinity of the nerves. At this point, nerve stimulation may be used to confirm accurate needle tip placement, or the anesthesiologist may rely on visualization alone to guide local anesthetic injection. Ultrasound imaging provides some distinct advantages, including the ability to avoid structures that a needle might damage (for instance, a blood vessel); fewer probing motions with the needle, which can be uncomfortable for patients; and direct observation of the site to deposit the local anesthetic solution, which improves accuracy and effectiveness of the block.

Table 7.4 Seven steps in a peripheral nerve block

1. Preoperative exam and obtaining anesthesia consent

2. Placement of monitors and positioning

3. Administration of intravenous sedation

4. Antibacterial skin preparation and numbing of skin

5. Use of localizing device (peripheral nerve stimulation or ultrasound)
   to detect nerve

6. Injection of local anesthetic solution

7. Brief pause for onset of nerve block before surgery

---

pain usually implies that the needle is in contact with the nerve and requires an adjustment of position. After the needle is in place, the injection
of medication should be pain-free; however, it is normal for you to feel
pressure at the site of injection.

When your anesthesiologist chooses to localize the peripheral nerve
with the nerve electrical stimulator method, he or she will first sedate you
and then apply antiseptic solution to your skin at the block site. You will
usually then receive an injection of a small dose of local anesthetic under
the skin where he or she will insert the needle (to reduce any discomfort).
The anesthesiologist will slowly insert the nerve block needle while the
peripheral nerve stimulator provides a short pulse of electrical energy to
the tip of the needle once or twice per second. As the needle approaches
your nerve, you will experience a rhythmic muscular movement of variable
intensity. Most people find the twitching sensation funny, odd, or mildly
unpleasant; some even laugh when they experience it because they are not
in control of their own movements. Few people find it painful.

If the needle bypasses the target nerve, or is too far from it, the muscle
twitch will diminish. The ability to see or feel this twitch, as currents on
the needle are dropped to a predetermined range, ensures that the needle
tip is close enough to the nerve to deposit local anesthetic and block nerve
transmission. Your anesthesiologist (or an assistant) will then inject the anesthetic agent—usually between 20 and 40 milliliters (1 to 3 tablespoons),
depending on the nerve blocked and the required duration of blockade. As
injection of the anesthetic begins, the twitching will stop. You will be asked
before or during injection to report any pain sensation or paresthesia below
the block site, which would indicate that the needle tip is too close to the

nerve fibers. If you have any such pain, the anesthesiologist will move the needle away from the nerve so that the injection can proceed safely.

When your anesthesiologist chooses to localize the peripheral nerve with the use of ultrasound imaging alone, he or she will inject the skin at the block site with local anesthetic after the nerve is localized. The anesthesiologist will then insert the block needle and guide it under direct observation to the nerve. The spread of the local anesthetic will be visible on the ultrasound image as it is injected around the nerve, and your anesthesiologist will move the needle short distances as necessary to ensure appropriate spread. If he or she chooses to use the nerve stimulation method in combination with ultrasound imaging to help localize the nerve, then you will experience muscle twitching as described above when the needle is brought close to the nerve. Anesthesiologists usually shut off the nerve stimulator at this point and use direct visualization to ensure correct placement of the local anesthetic.

When your anesthesiologist injects the local anesthetic at the appropriate place, you will experience numbness, heaviness, warmth, and clumsiness of your limb (blocks in the nerves of the trunk usually produce only numbness). Eventually, you will completely lose strength and sensation in the distribution of the nerves that were blocked. Numbness can occur almost immediately or may evolve over 20 to 30 minutes, depending on how quickly the drug makes its way across the protective sheaths encompassing the nerve and into the nerve fibers. This time of onset varies among individuals. In addition, there may be differences in individual susceptibility to the drugs used.

Anesthesiologists usually perform blocks before surgery begins, although they may also perform them afterward when the patient is in the recovery area. Performing blocks after surgery is challenging because adopting positions necessary for the nerve block may be difficult or impossible for patients, and because splints, braces, and bandages may be in the way. In addition, patients who have undergone surgery have been sedated and given pain medication in the recovery area and therefore may not be able to legally give consent for a nerve block. When anesthesiologists perform blocks in the recovery room after surgery, it is usually because the surgery produced more pain than was expected. In some such cases, intravenous medications may be insufficient to provide the desired pain relief, and a nerve block can provide a major improvement in pain control.

You may be hesitant, like many surgical patients, to undergo peripheral nerve blocks because of the perception that they will be very painful. However, as with neuraxial blocks, the combination of local anesthetic injected in the skin before the block and a modest amount of sedation generally make the experience no more unpleasant than having an IV inserted. If the procedure does cause pain, tell your anesthesiologist so that he or she can help alleviate it. Pain control may require more local anesthetic at the site of the block, more sedation, or a change in needle position, but it can usually be accomplished quickly. Patients who have undergone nerve blocks to help reduce postoperative pain are usually very satisfied with the technique. Several studies have shown a higher degree of satisfaction with peripheral nerve blockade in the anesthetic plan than with general anesthesia alone followed by opioid drugs to relieve pain.

Peripheral nerve blocks can be used alone to provide anesthesia for some surgeries, or in combination with sedation, neuraxial (spinal) anesthesia, or general anesthesia (table 7.5). There are many advantages of using peripheral nerve blocks instead of other types of anesthesia. Whereas general anesthesia will make you unconscious and usually requires you to have a breathing tube of some sort, a small amount of sedation in conjunction with a peripheral nerve block will merely put you in a light sleep. If you tell your anesthesiologist that you would rather be more asleep after he or she has already administered sedative medication, this can be addressed readily with additional medication. Thus, sedation can often be tailored to the desire of the patient. Another important advantage of peripheral nerve blocks is that patients will be relatively comfortable after surgery instead of experiencing the intense pain that may occur after awakening from surgery conducted with general anesthesia alone. This is especially true for patients who undergo markedly painful procedures, such as those involving bones or joints.

Peripheral nerve blocks can be used in many different areas of the body and for many different types of surgeries, such as eye surgery (an ophthalmologist often performs this type of block), upper or lower extremity surgery, and breast or hernia surgery. At some hospitals, anesthesiologists even use peripheral nerve blockade for carotid artery surgery in the neck. Peripheral nerve blocks are most often used for orthopedic surgery, which focuses on the extremities and can involve significant and lasting pain because incisions are made in the joints, bones, and ligaments. If you are undergoing an orthopedic procedure, you may choose to be unconscious with general anesthesia and to receive morphine injections during and after recovery

Table 7.5 **Uses of peripheral nerve blockade**

Stand-alone anesthetic (with patient awake), per patient request or for very ill patients

Combined with sedation, for a light plane of unconsciousness

Combined with neuraxial (spinal) anesthetic, usually with sedation

Combined with general anesthesia

---

from anesthesia. However, the integration of nerve blocks into your anesthesia management plan creates several other anesthesia possibilities for you to consider. For example, a nerve block that completely numbs the surgical area can stand alone as its own anesthetic, with no additional medication whatsoever. On the other hand, if you are like most patients and prefer to be asleep, your anesthesiologist could also administer sedation along with such a block to make you comfortable and help control your anxiety. For lower extremity procedures, the neuraxial nerve blocks discussed in the last chapter offer yet another possible anesthetic choice.

A nerve block that provides excellent pain relief from surgical incisions may not be adequate to provide complete anesthesia during your orthopedic surgery. In this case, your anesthesiologist can still use the peripheral nerve block as an integral part of the anesthetic. He or she will then use general or spinal anesthesia in combination with the nerve block in the operating room. For example, peripheral blocks may not be adequate for surgery that involves the use of a pneumatic tourniquet on the arm or leg that is inflated to relatively high pressures. The tourniquet reduces blood loss and vastly improves visibility for the surgeon, but it can be quite uncomfortable for the patient over time. The addition of peripheral nerve blockade to general or spinal anesthesia in such a case is beneficial in providing postoperative pain relief and helping the patient make the transition from the operating room to PACU, and eventually to the hospital bed (or home). Peripheral nerve blocks may also help you during rehabilitation, especially when administered as continuous infusions by nerve block catheters over several days.

If you are undergoing surgery with spinal anesthesia, peripheral nerve blockade can extend the duration of the spinal block, as well as providing longer-term control of your postoperative pain. If you are undergoing surgery with general anesthesia, a pre-existing peripheral block typically reduces the amount of anesthetic necessary for you to be comfortable and unconscious, which in turn allows you to wake up more easily, feeling more comfortable, with a reduced need for opioid pain medications (and therefore minimizing or avoiding their many side effects).

In the case of surgery involving the head, neck, and arm, peripheral nerve blocks are especially useful. It is difficult for anesthesiologists to use neuraxial regional anesthesia (spinal or epidural blocks) safely in these areas because inserting the needle high in the spine endangers the spinal cord, which is tightly constrained in the cervical (neck) region. Although anesthesiologists can perform cervical (neck) epidural blocks, they are most safely performed with x-ray guidance in a fluoroscopy suite, and are therefore not common in operative anesthesia in the United States.

The benefits of peripheral nerve blocks in surgery of the lower extremity may not be quite so obvious to you. In terms of pain relief, epidural blocks can be just as effective as peripheral nerve blocks in surgeries of the legs or lower trunk. Because some major lower extremity orthopedic procedures require two sites of peripheral nerve blockade and catheter insertion for continuous postoperative pain relief (to anesthetize nerves coming out of the two different nerve plexuses that go to each leg), epidural blocks may seem simpler and less uncomfortable for the patient. However, there are several side effects and potential complications of neuraxial regional anesthesia (table 7.6) that must be considered. Some patients cannot tolerate the diminished blood pressures associated with epidural and spinal blocks. Blood pressure issues can increase the intensity of nursing and may require observation in a critical care unit, which is inconvenient for patients and families and can dramatically increase the costs of the hospitalization. Another complication involved with epidural or spinal blocks, which we explore in greater detail in the next chapter, is the possibility of hemorrhage into the spinal canal. Patients who are on blood-thinning or anticoagulation medications, which orthopedic surgeons increasingly use to prevent postoperative clots, may be at a significantly higher risk for such hemorrhage.

An additional factor is that spinal and epidural blocks almost always affect both legs of the patient, whereas peripheral nerve blockade only affects one. Therefore, a patient's abilities to get out of bed, ambulate with a brace or crutches, and participate actively in physical therapy can be markedly enhanced after orthopedic surgery with the use of peripheral nerve blockade. Studies comparing peripheral nerve blockade and epidural blocks for pain control after major lower extremity orthopedic surgeries have shown

Table 7.6 Potential advantages of peripheral nerve blocks instead of neuraxial blocks

---

No risk of spinal hematoma or of injury to spinal cord

Less invasive and potentially less painful

No blood pressure compromise

No risk of urine retention

No itching (often seen with spinal or epidural blocks if opioids are used for postoperative pain)

Only one leg affected in lower extremity surgeries (reduces fall risk)

---

that, although pain relief is similar with the two modalities, fewer undesirable side effects occur with peripheral blocks than with epidural blocks.

Peripheral nerve blockade is not without its own potential adverse effects (table 7.7). Patients may experience discomfort at the site of injection during and after the block, but this is usually minor. When arteries or veins are close to the nerve being blocked, small amounts of bleeding can occur and contribute to soreness. In addition, the feeling of a numb, heavy, and clumsy limb after a peripheral nerve block can be disturbing to some people, although most consider it the lesser of two evils when compared to the pain after surgery. Precautions must be taken to avoid damaging a numb limb for the duration of the nerve block because patients can't register normal pain or discomfort, the warning signs of injury.

Nerve blocks that do not involve placement of catheters last 4 to 12 hours but can be prolonged up to 24 hours when certain additives are included with the local anesthetic solution. Your doctor or nurse will give you instructions for care and avoidance of injury after a peripheral nerve block when you are discharged from the hospital or ambulatory care center. If you've had surgery on the upper half of your body, you will usually have a sling or shoulder immobilizer. For lower extremity surgery, your affected leg may remain weak and numb at the time of discharge, in which case your doctor's main concerns will be injury and the risk of falling. You should not bear weight on a blocked leg until your strength completely returns. Your provider will train you in the use of crutches so that you will

Table 7.7 **Potential side effects of peripheral nerve blocks**

Pain at site

Bleeding at site, hematoma

Numb limb for 8–72 hours (depending on whether continuous catheter is used)

Prolonged tingling or numbness in up to 14% of patients

Weakness that could lead to fall (lower extremity blocks)

---

be comfortable using them until the numbness and weakness resolve. In addition, he or she may give you a brace to add support for the duration of the block (this is most common after knee surgery).

As your block begins to wear off, you may feel a tingling sensation that can be unpleasant but is normal. Most clinicians encourage patients to start taking their oral pain medications (usually prescribed by their surgeon) as soon as there is any evidence of resolution of the block (such as tingling or the onset of surgical pain), or even while the block is still in place, toward the end of its expected duration. This allows a transition to the use of the oral pain medication, which will help you avoid the development of severe incision pain. It is generally easier to "stay ahead" of the pain with active management than to attempt to "catch up" to it when it has been allowed to become fully developed.

Many side effects that are experienced with general anesthesia do not typically occur with peripheral nerve blockade. Nausea, the most common and one of the most dreaded complications of general anesthesia, occurs much less often when nerve blocks are a component of the anesthetic plan. In fact, anesthesiologists at outpatient surgery centers emphasize the inclusion of peripheral nerve blockade whenever possible to avoid general anesthesia and reduce the need for postoperative injections of opioid medications for pain control. These actions dramatically reduce nausea, shorten the hospital stay, and reduce the frequency of unplanned hospital admissions—all effects that increase patient satisfaction. The lethargy, sleepiness, and prolonged mental compromise that many people experience with general anesthesia are typically avoided or minimized when peripheral nerve blockade is the primary anesthetic, even though sedation is often used with the block to keep patients asleep throughout the procedure.

A patient who has undergone surgery with regional anesthesia (with or without sedation) will appear very different in the recovery room from a patient who has undergone the same procedure with general anesthesia. The patient who had a regional block will usually be much more alert, relatively comfortable, and be able to sit up, communicate, and leave the recovery area (and the hospital) sooner. The patient who had general anesthesia will often be very sleepy, and when awakened, will complain of incisional pain that requires administration of intravenous morphine or another potent opioid. These drugs frequently cause nausea, which may lead to the use of additional sedating medications to help the patient cope with this adverse effect. Having seen the difference in two such scenarios, I believe that many patients who opt for general anesthesia alone would be more comfortable and satisfied in the postoperative period if some form of regional anesthesia were integrated into their anesthetic plan.

Chapter 8

Complications of Regional Anesthesia

 What are the most common complications of regional anesthesia?

What happens if the needle hits a blood vessel during a nerve block?

What are the risks associated with blood thinners and nerve blocks?

Can the site of a nerve block become infected?

How common are nerve injuries during nerve block procedures? Are they permanent?

What are the symptoms of a nerve injury from a nerve block?

What happens if I have a reaction to the local anesthetic?

How do anesthesiologists avoid patient reactions to local anesthetic?

Anesthesiologists sometimes use regional anesthesia rather than general anesthesia to avoid certain risks and complications of general anesthesia, such as difficult airway issues, dental injuries, postoperative nausea, or major cardiovascular or respiratory disturbances, or simply because it is the preferred anesthetic method in a given setting. In many other situations, regional techniques are used *with* general anesthesia to provide improved pain control and to reduce the amount of anesthetics and opioids needed.

Table 8.1 Possible severe complications of regional anesthesia blocks (for both neuraxial and peripheral blocks)

Bleeding at site of injection

Hematoma at site of injection

Spinal hematoma (with spinal or epidural blocks)

Infection at injection site

Spinal infection: meningitis or abscess (with spinal or epidural blocks)

Nerve injury (loss of sensation, weakness)

Nerve dysfunction (numbness, tingling)

Allergic reactions to local anesthetic drugs

Local anesthetic toxicity to nervous system (confusion, tremor, seizure in extreme cases)

Local anesthetic toxicity to cardiovascular system (blood pressure reduction, heart rhythm disturbances, cardiac arrest in extreme cases)

Cardiac arrest with spinal anesthetic (due to "high spinal" effect)

Transient neurologic syndrome with spinal blocks (back pain, may radiate to legs)

Although many complications of general anesthesia can be avoided with regional techniques, regional anesthesia has its own potential risks and hazards (table 8.1).

If you will be undergoing regional anesthesia, first you should be aware of the complications that can occur with any needle injection—bleeding and infection. Minor bleeding beneath the skin is common with injections and usually appears only as a bruise, although there may be slight tenderness in that spot for several days. More significant bleeding, called a *hematoma*, is the result of blood leaking from a blood vessel. Hematomas are more prominent and painful than simple bruises, but they heal spontaneously over time as the body reabsorbs the blood. With regional anesthetic techniques, hematomas are most likely to occur when a blood vessel, particularly an artery, is located directly adjacent to a nerve.

If an anesthesiologist inserts the needle through an artery to locate the nerve, then the patient is more likely to develop a hematoma. This ap-

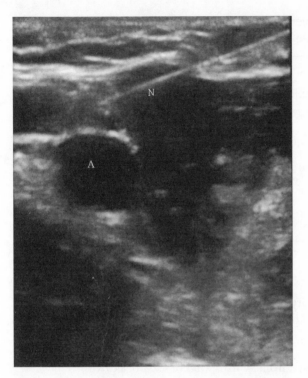

Figure 8.1 A still photograph of the ultrasound image that the anesthesiologist observes during an ultrasound-guided nerve block. In this case, the block is in the axilla, or armpit, and will block the nerves to the lower arm and hand. The nerves lie in close proximity to the blood vessels in this region. The anesthesiologist conducts the nerve block while observing the ultrasound pictures in real time, which means that he or she watches the needle continuously during insertion and observes the spread of the local anesthetic solution. In this image, the shaft of the needle (N) is seen as a straight white line; its proximity to the axillary artery (A) is closely monitored to avoid perforating the blood vessel while delivering local anesthetic adjacent to the nerves.

proach used to be common in upper extremity nerve blocks for forearm and hand surgery. It is still used today by some anesthesiologists, although the peripheral nerve stimulator and ultrasound methods of localization have become more common; either of these reduces the likelihood of inserting the needle into a vessel (figure 8.1). In large studies evaluating the risks of upper extremity blocks in which the needle was placed through the artery, the rate of significant bleeding-related complications was very low (about 1 in 1,000 cases). Other blood-related complications of blocks involving a needle placed through the artery include swelling, pain, and spasm (constriction) of the blood vessel.

Whereas significant bleeding complications of peripheral nerve blockade are rare and seldom serious, neuraxial (spinal and epidural) techniques carry a higher risk of bleeding in certain situations. Insertion of a needle into the spinal canal results in trauma to small veins or arteries in the epidural space; anesthesiologists commonly see drops of blood in the spinal fluid or in the epidural needle during this procedure. However, the body's normal blood-clotting mechanisms generally prevent this minor trauma from leading to a hematoma in the spine.

When blood does collect in the spine, especially under the pressure created by injury to a small artery, it can lead to irreversible damage to the spinal cord or the nerve roots. Many orthopedic surgeons today prescribe blood-thinning medications before and/or after surgery (an often life-saving intervention) to reduce their patients' likelihood of developing postoperative clots. Patients taking these medications and undergoing neuraxial regional anesthesia, especially epidural blocks, are at an increased risk of a spinal hematoma (figure 8.2). Such hematomas can be difficult to recognize because they are not always painful, and the weakness they cause in the legs can be confused with the effects of the epidural itself. If surgeons do not act rapidly to treat the bleeding, preferably within 12 hours, patients may have permanent lower extremity nerve injury, even paralysis. The American Society of Regional Anesthesia and Pain Medicine issued guidelines, most recently in 2010, for anesthesiologists on how to safely use neuraxial anesthesia techniques with patients who are taking blood-thinning medications. The use of these guidelines is intended to significantly reduce the risk of intraspinal bleeding related to needle insertion and epidural catheter insertion and removal.

The other notable complication of needle injections is infection. Anesthesiologists perform nerve blocks under sterile conditions (cleaning and preparing the skin and using sterile gloves and instruments), so infection is extraordinarily rare after single-injection procedures. When a catheter is inserted as part of a patient's anesthesia plan, and maintained for several days, bacterial contamination is more likely. In studies of various types of nerve block catheters, between one-fourth and one-half of the catheters from heavily contaminated skin areas (such as the groin) were found to

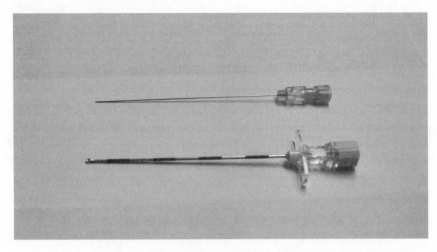

Figure 8.2 A spinal needle (top) and an epidural needle (bottom). Both are placed within the spine after the skin and deeper tissues are anesthetized with local anesthetic. The larger bore of the epidural needle presents a higher risk of traumatizing a blood vessel within the spine. Further, the insertion of a small, plastic, flexible catheter through the large needle (and later removing it), increases the risk of bleeding compared with the spinal block.

be colonized with bacteria within 48 hours. However, only a tiny fraction of patients with these catheters had any signs of true infection, and many who did were effectively treated simply by removing the catheter. Because nerve block catheters are typically in place for only a short time (usually two to three days), infectious complications are very unusual. Likewise, spinal infection after neuraxial regional anesthesia is also extremely rare (1 case in 10,000 to 30,000), unless an epidural catheter is left in place for a prolonged period.

Along with bleeding and infection, injuring a nerve during a block procedure is one of your anesthesiologist's greatest concerns. As discussed in chapter 6, a *paresthesia* is the sensation a person feels when the sensory portion of a nerve is contacted. Most paresthesias that occur during regional anesthesia are temporary and harmless. Although some studies have suggested that nerve injuries related to regional anesthesia are preceded by paresthesias, the relationship is not yet clear. Other studies have not revealed an increased incidence of nerve injury after paresthesia, even when anesthesiologists deliberately use these sensations to guide nerve blocks. Most paresthesias are not associated with any neurological injury, but even so, the majority of anesthesiologists have stopped using the paresthesia technique to locate peripheral nerves. Even with electrical nerve locators, or the use of ultrasound guidance, nerve injuries can occur. And it is clear that nerve injury can occur without the patient ever having sensed a paresthesia.

All this adds up to continued uncertainty about the cause of nerve injury during regional anesthesia. Nerve injuries also occur during general anesthesia, where pressure on the nerve or stretching of the nerve for prolonged periods can decrease blood flow to the delicate fibers inside. The result can be nerve fiber dysfunction or nerve fiber destruction, which may be evident immediately or may take days to become apparent. After general anesthesia, some patients have normal nerve function in the recovery room but develop a weakness or numbness over the next several days, which is likely evidence of a nerve injury. Certain body positions required for surgery (such as lying on one side, or having the legs elevated in stirrups), as well as low blood pressure and significant blood loss, are known to increase the chance that a patient will develop nerve injuries during general anesthesia.

Although the exact causes of nerve injury during regional anesthesia are not yet clear, researchers have identified several contributors to these injuries, including high concentrations of local anesthetic, repeated blind injections of the same nerve to improve an inadequate or incomplete nerve block, the shape of the needle used for blocking, and, in particular, injection of medication directly into a nerve *fascicle* (a bundle of microscopic nerve fibers that course within the outer protective membrane of the peripheral nerve). Anesthesiologists are alerted to the possibility of injection into a nerve fascicle when the patient feels a paresthesia in the area that the nerve innervates as injection begins or when higher than usual pressure must be applied on the syringe to inject the solution during the block. Ultrasound imaging during the block can also alert a practitioner about the potential for injection into the nerve fascicle.

The best way for anesthesiologists to ensure low rates of nerve injury during regional anesthesia is for them to closely adhere to patient safety guidelines. These guidelines include using the lowest practical concentration of local anesthetic, avoiding nerve trauma with the needle (or catheter), injecting slowly and gently to avoid forcing medication into a nerve fascicle, and making certain that needle placement is not too close to the nerve (through the use of electronic nerve stimulation and/or ultrasound guidance). Patients whose nerves have significant pre-existing damage may be more susceptible to injury during the block or injection process, so the physician will need to carefully weigh the need for a block in these patients. As with any medical procedure, individual physician judgment is important.

Because high concentrations of otherwise safe local anesthetic medications can be injurious to nerves, such injury is most likely a function of both time and concentration (that is, longer exposure increases the chance of toxicity). For this reason, continuous infusions of local anesthetic through peripheral nerve catheters or epidural catheters usually contain very low concentrations of the drug. The low doses are adequate for catheter use because controlling incision pain after surgery requires less numbness than anesthetizing a limb for surgery. Furthermore, this partial degree of block allows patients to move their extremities after surgery.

❋ How likely are you to experience a nerve injury if you undergo a nerve block procedure? Estimates of nerve injury vary from as low as .03 percent up to 14 percent, depending on how researchers define injury, the type of block, the study population, and the method of data collection. For example, when researchers interview patients using questions that have a specific focus on neurological function, complications are more evident than if they simply wait for feedback from the patients or surgeons involved. Studies that show higher rates of postoperative nerve dysfunction demonstrate minor degrees of sensory loss, which typically heals spontaneously in days to a few weeks.

When anesthesiologists use regional anesthesia techniques for orthopedic surgery, it can be difficult to tell whether nerve injury is a result of the surgical procedure, the nerve block, or something unrelated, such as positioning of the extremity or use of a tourniquet (table 8.2). Surgery alone without regional anesthesia is associated with a certain degree of complications, including nerve injury. In addition, in some situations regional anesthesia and surgical factors both contribute to nerve injury.

The risk of nerve injuries should not be understated. However, it should be comforting to know that such injuries usually show up as areas of numbness or tingling, instead of muscle weakness or paralysis. In addition, most heal after a few days or weeks without any specific therapy. More severe (and rare) nerve injuries, which involve dense areas of sensory loss or deficits in muscle function, may take months to heal as the nerves slowly regenerate. Diagnosing severe nerve injuries can be difficult because it is

Table 8.2   Possible causes of nerve injury during surgery

Regional anesthesia block

needle injury

high-pressure injection

toxicity to nerve from local anesthetic drugs

Surgical and anesthetic manipulations

pressure-related positioning injury (pressure over nerve for long period)

stretch of nerves from adverse positioning (reduced blood flow to nerves)

use of surgical tourniquet at high pressure or for a prolonged period (reduced blood flow to nerves)

incision affecting small skin nerves (unavoidable)

retraction of tissues with surgical instruments, which presses on small nerves

sharp or blunt injury to deeper local nerves

Postoperative influences

local inflammation affecting small nerves

swelling with compression of nerves at incision area and in distal parts of the upper or lower extremities

constriction from immobilizing devices on extremities: casts, splints, wraps, braces (pressure on nerves; worsens with swelling)

aggressive physical therapy for previously underused extremities may unmask or predispose to compressed, or "pinched," nerves

hard to pinpoint the area of a sensory nerve injury, and what has occurred to damage the nerve fibers is not always clear. When patients who have sustained an apparent nerve injury do not improve after several weeks, many anesthesiologists or surgeons refer them to a neurologist physical medicine specialist for further evaluation.

Compromised nerve function sometimes occurs after orthopedic surgery because of the postoperative swelling, splinting, and active rehabilitation and physical therapy that follow this kind of surgery. For instance, in patients who have had shoulder surgery, nerve injuries may be the result of processes that are not related to the operation or to the anesthetic block. These conditions include carpal tunnel syndrome (nerve compression at the wrist) and nerve entrapment behind the elbow. Some patients are predisposed to these "pinched nerve" conditions, which are sometimes made worse by surgery and the recovery process. In a recent large-scale study, significant nerve injuries after surgery conducted with peripheral nerve blockade occurred in approximately 1 out of 1,000 cases, but after careful evaluation, it was noted that only about 10 percent of the injuries were actually related to the nerve block procedure.

In addition, a major study from the Mayo Clinic has provided strong evidence that inclusion of peripheral nerve blockade with one of the most commonly performed orthopedic surgeries, total knee replacement, does not increase the risk of nerve injury. The authors evaluated their computerized database, encompassing more than 19,000 cases over two decades, and found that the inclusion of nerve blocks for pain control as a complement to the primary anesthetic (either general anesthesia or spinal anesthesia) increased dramatically over this period, from very few to over 85 percent of cases. Despite this tremendous expansion in the use of nerve blocks at this institution, there was no increase in the frequency of nerve injury during this time, a testament to the safety of these techniques.

Local anesthetic medications themselves can also be harmful to patients. Allergy to these medications is unusual but possible. Many so-called "allergic" responses to procaine (Novocain) or lidocaine are actually adverse effects of adrenaline, which is often mixed with these drugs to help prolong the duration of the block. Patients frequently report palpitations, dizziness, and the feeling of being faint after an injection of Novocain into the mouth. True allergies are more likely to cause difficulty breathing, rash, or a severe drop in blood pressure and will require specific medical treatment. On the other hand, the side effects of adrenaline subside in a few minutes as long as no further medication is injected. In the past, preservative agents were added to anesthetic medications to help them last longer on the shelf, and it was these preservatives that often caused actual allergic responses in patients. Preservatives in anesthetic drugs are much less prevalent today.

Local anesthetics can produce other types of toxicity aside from allergic reactions. As with any medication, the injection of too high a dose can cause adverse effects. The level of dosage depends on where the drug is placed, the rate of injection, and whether the drug will reach vulnerable structures or organs. Deciding on the amount of medication to give a patient is more complex than merely administering a dose according to the patient's body weight. Although anesthesiologists are familiar with recommended maximal doses of local anesthetics, these data are derived primarily from animal laboratory studies, and they are only a guide to what would constitute an overdose. In fact, even a very small dose can produce toxic effects if it rapidly gains access to susceptible organs or tissues—in particular, the brain or the heart. On the other hand, physicians sometimes use much larger doses of local anesthetic when the likelihood of absorption is very small, such as when plastic surgeons inject lidocaine into fat planes to reduce the pain of liposuction.

When local anesthetic medication is injected, it acts on nerves in the area to block nerve conduction and thus provide pain relief. If the medication is confined to the tissues next to the nerve, the risk of toxicity is extremely low. While the injection is being given, however, drugs can inadvertently gain access to small blood vessels or lymphatic channels, resulting in high blood levels and toxicity. Furthermore, blood vessels in the area of injection may absorb the anesthetic at variable rates, again resulting in potential toxicity.

Toxic effects produced by local anesthetics fall into two broad groups: toxicity to the central nervous system, which is most common, and toxicity to the cardiovascular system. When the central nervous system is exposed to local anesthetics, patients may experience minor symptoms of toxicity, including twitching, confusion, loss of coordination, visual changes, and other unusual sensory perceptions, such as metallic tastes in the mouth, numbness around the mouth or lips, or ringing or roaring in the ears. More severe toxic effects include seizure. These symptoms are generally brief and temporary, and they usually end before any treatment is necessary. If a seizure persists, physicians can use medications that are readily available in anesthetizing areas and operating rooms to stop the seizure within seconds. Patients will not remember this occurrence, and surgery can proceed as planned, as long as all symptoms of local anesthetic toxicity have gone away and the patient, surgeon, and family wish to continue. Toxic reactions usually occur immediately upon injection of the local anesthetic, but they can occur minutes or even an hour later. These reactions are not related to epilepsy and do not make the patient more vulnerable to subsequent seizures or central nervous system injury.

A more serious and much rarer type of local anesthetic toxicity affects the heart. Toxicity to the cardiovascular system occurs when local anesthetics gain rapid access to the bloodstream, because they are either inadvertently injected into a vessel or rapidly absorbed into the bloodstream. Symptoms include abnormal heart rhythms, severe falls in blood pressure, and even cardiac arrest. The threat of such reactions prompted members of the pharmaceutical industry to create newer and less toxic agents. Two such local anesthetic drugs, levobupivacaine and ropivacaine, were introduced in the late 1990s and appeared in laboratory research to be less toxic to the cardiovascular system than older medications. These drugs are now widely available, and the older, more toxic, agents are used less often. Recent research into the causes and treatment of cardiovascular toxicity from local anesthetics has led to the development of a new therapy that has been useful in several cases of severe cardiac toxicity. This injection of intravenous lipid emulsion to "absorb" the excess local anesthetic molecules has proved to be truly life saving.

Local anesthetic medications may become blood-borne during or after injection with any type of regional anesthesia technique, including the spinal block, epidural block, and peripheral nerve block. The likelihood of toxicity is much lower during spinal blocks than during epidural blocks because the dose of drug is very low, and because the spinal needle penetrates the dural sac, which does not contain blood vessels of any significant size. Even in the case of peripheral nerve blocks or epidural blocks, which involve higher local anesthetic doses, toxicity is extremely unlikely and occurs in approximately 1 in 1,000 to 3,000 cases. As anesthesiologists use ultrasound guidance more often with regional anesthesia care, allowing visualization of blood vessels, more precise needle tip placement, and lower doses of local anesthetic, the likelihood of toxicity should decrease even more.

Spinal nerve blocks may also result in a different type of toxicity—one that is based on the rapid interruption of nerve function as the anesthetic affects the nerve roots. On rare occasions, the influence (or level) of a spinal block may extend much higher in the body than the anesthesiologist expects. This unexpected occurrence could be the result of pressure waves in the fluid inside the dural sac, or because of the widely varying volumes of this sac fluid among individuals. When a block ascends to high levels, not only does it cause blood vessels in the legs and lower body to relax (dropping the patient's blood pressure), but it also may affect nerves that supply the heart, which are an essential part of the reflex response that compensates for the drop in blood pressure. Instead of an acceleration of the heart rate and an increase in the force of pumping to eject more blood, the heart is unable to compensate. This lack of compensation may lead to further falls in blood pressure, setting up a life-threatening sequence of events in which reduced blood flow causes even worsening heart function, and eventually all circulation ceases. The anesthesiologist must recognize the situation and intervene to interrupt this cycle before it becomes too advanced; practitioners are trained to be vigilant for this situation, called a *high spinal*, which causes a very low blood pressure and possibly even cardiac arrest, during spinal nerve blocks. Fortunately, high spinal is rare; most practicing anesthesiologists will encounter it only a few times in their entire careers.

Sometimes a high spinal level will cause primarily respiratory instead of cardiac symptoms. Because higher levels of spinal block may weaken the respiratory muscles, patients may develop shortness of breath and require assistance with breathing and other measures to help stabilize the blood pressure while the spinal block level descends, which is often just a matter of minutes. As with the toxicity from peripheral nerve blocks discussed earlier in the chapter, such reactions are very uncommon. Elderly patients with severe underlying diseases are most likely to develop respiratory symptoms from high spinal blocks.

Epidural blocks can also rise to high levels of the body, causing respiratory compromise and deterioration of cardiovascular function. However, these complications are more common with spinal blockade because of the rapid onset of spinal anesthesia and the injection of all medication at one time during the block. Some peripheral nerve blocks placed near the spine, such as an *interscalene block* for shoulder surgery or a *lumbar plexus block* for major hip or knee surgery, can also (rarely) result in cardiovascular and respiratory consequences. Careful needle placement, slow injection, thorough knowledge of the anatomy, and frequent communication between the anesthesiologist and the patient during the block greatly decrease the risk of these complications.

Another potentially toxic effect of spinal anesthetics is *transient neurologic syndrome* (TNS). This condition varies in severity from mild back discomfort to severe pain in the lower back. It may also cause pain that radiates into the legs, muscle weakness, or sensory loss in the lower extremities. The most common medication-related cause of TNS is lidocaine, a spinal anesthetic for short surgical cases. Although most TNS cases involve back pain without any compromise of neurological function, this syndrome has practically ended the use of lidocaine in spinal anesthesia. The substitution of other local anesthetics for short-acting spinal blockade has resulted in a marked decline in the incidence of TNS.

❀ The most significant factor in safe regional anesthesia is the anesthesiologist's understanding of which patients are at risk and should not be anesthetized by certain techniques. Regional anesthesia involves needles near vulnerable structures, injections of potentially toxic substances, the loss of strength and sensation, and effects on the respiratory and cardiovascular systems. As a result, under certain recognized conditions in specific patients, regional blocks should not be used. These conditions are different for peripheral nerve blockade and for neuraxial regional anesthesia. Patients with such conditions, who therefore cannot receive regional anesthesia techniques, will nonetheless benefit from an injection of local anesthesia at the incision site, along with sedation or general anesthesia, for their surgical procedures. Postoperative pain in these patients must be controlled by other methods, including intravenous injections of opioids, nonopioid pain medications, and patient-controlled anesthesia (PCA) pumps.

❀ You should understand the risks of regional anesthesia techniques before providing consent for this type of anesthesia. Serious side effects or complications are rare, however, and will probably be even rarer in the future. The many benefits of regional anesthesia techniques appear to outweigh the risks for most patients. Careful physician judgment is imperative in identifying patients who should not receive regional anesthetic blocks, and ensuring a high degree of safety for those who do.

Chapter 9

Regional Anesthesia for Special Populations

 Why do anesthesiologists usually place regional anesthetic blocks in children only after general anesthesia has been initiated?

Are nerve blocks safe to use in children under general anesthesia?

How can regional blocks benefit children who are undergoing surgery?

How has ultrasound affected the practice of pediatric regional anesthesia?

What are the risks of using general anesthesia during labor and delivery?

What are the benefits of using spinal or epidural blocks during labor and delivery?

Why is the epidural block the preferred anesthetic for women in labor?

How do epidural blocks affect labor, delivery, and the likelihood of a cesarean section?

What other regional anesthesia methods are sometimes used in labor and delivery?

Why does general anesthesia pose special risks to people with obstructive sleep apnea?

What are the disadvantages of opioid pain medications for patients with sleep apnea?

What are the benefits of regional anesthesia for patients with sleep apnea who undergo surgery?

What is the impact of general anesthesia and opioid pain medications on brain function in the elderly?

Can the use of regional blocks in the elderly lead to an improvement in postoperative complication rates?

Children

Nerve blocks and regional anesthesia are just as useful in children as they are in adults. Children pose special challenges to anesthesiologists, however. They are emotionally immature, are naturally afraid of any painful procedure, and are not able to understand the benefit of medical procedures. A physician must keep in mind the special nature of children and decide how to interact with a particular child when planning anesthesia.

Although it is more difficult to utilize regional anesthesia techniques in a frightened child, they can help the anesthesiologist provide more effective pain control and can reduce the amount of anesthetic medications necessary in the operating room. Regional anesthesia has the same beneficial effects in children as in adults: postoperative anesthetic side effects are reduced, comfort and satisfaction are improved, and patients and parents can usually leave the hospital sooner than if general anesthesia alone (with higher doses of opioid medications) is used for surgery.

In fact, when regional techniques are incorporated into pediatric anesthesia, some procedures that would ordinarily require admitting the child to the hospital for pain control may instead be done on an outpatient basis, and the child can go home the same day. Furthermore, some infants, particularly those born prematurely, are at significant risk for postoperative *apnea* (failure to breathe) due to the effect of anesthetics and pain medications. Anesthesiologists can decrease the risk of infant apnea by incorporating regional blocks into the anesthesia plan, both in the operating room and in the recovery process, and therefore avoiding opioid medications that would increase the risk of apnea in the very young infant.

Many of the same regional blocks used for adults can be used in children and infants, but they may have to be used in a different fashion. For example, anesthesiologists often place blocks in pediatric patients after general anesthesia has been started because children are not able to tolerate pain or communicate effectively during neuraxial blocks or peripheral nerve blocks. Adults are usually sedated when regional blocks are performed, but they are aware enough of the procedure to communicate with the anesthesiologist. The communication makes the anesthesiologist immediately aware of contact with the nerves, and the anesthesiologist can then alter the needle path accordingly. Communication between anesthesiologist and patient is a basic principle of regional anesthesia; the exceptions include children and anyone who is uncontrollable or uncooperative. When anesthesiologists determine that the benefits of regional techniques outweigh any risk of placing local anesthetics near nerves in unconscious patients, it is acceptable for them to proceed with placement of nerve blocks under general anesthesia.

Of the different types of regional anesthesia, spinal blocks specifically benefit pediatric patients with respiratory problems such as premature infants with lung disorders or abnormalities of breathing control that result in apnea. Children with serious lung disorders, such as cystic fibrosis or severe asthma, may also benefit if breathing tubes and mechanical ventilation, which are common with general anesthesia, can be avoided. Spinal blocks can sometimes be used instead of general anesthesia in such patients. To take advantage of the preserved natural airway and normal breathing pattern, anesthesiologists usually provide the infant or child with a small amount of sedation and then place spinal blocks in the awake patient.

On the other hand, anesthesiologists usually place epidural blocks and catheters in small children after general anesthesia has been administered. For the anesthesiologist to find the epidural space by sense of feel requires the patient to be absolutely still. As with adults, epidurals can be placed in children at lumbar levels, for procedures involving the lower extremities, groin, or lower abdominal areas, or at thoracic levels, for surgery involving the upper abdomen or chest. The epidural catheter is useful for infusing pain-controlling local anesthetics and opioids for days after the procedure. Although not yet firmly established, the use of ultrasound in placing blocks and catheters in children is gaining popularity among anesthesiologists.

A third type of neuraxial block that anesthesiologists use in infants and young children is the *caudal* block. Although this technique was once used for women in labor, it is seldom used in adults today, probably because the epidural block is more versatile. The caudal block takes advantage of certain anatomic features of young children. In this procedure, the anesthesiologist inserts the needle at the very bottom of the spine (at the upper part of the cleft between the buttocks) after general anesthesia has been initiated.

The patient is held on his or her side, and the bottom part of the spinal canal, called the *caudal canal*, is located by pressing in the buttocks cleft. This space is the lowest portion of the bony canal in which the spinal cord is situated. The anesthesiologist can inject the local anesthetic safely at this level because the spinal cord (and its protective dural sac) ends higher in the spine. The caudal canal contains only the lowest nerve roots that run to the groin and anal area. An injection at this level will affect these and higher nerve roots, and patients who undergo procedures after this type of block will have minimal pain for the first 12 to 24 hours after surgery. Although this is not anatomically feasible in adults, anesthesiologists can easily place catheters in the caudal canal in most young children, providing several days of inpatient pain control with an infusion of medication. The caudal block is much like a low epidural block and is most often used in children undergoing hernia repair and surgery on the genital region.

Peripheral nerve blockade is not as frequently used in children as in adults, but it is being used more and more commonly in pediatric centers. Anesthesiologists may use penile blocks in children for the pain of circumcision, ilio-inguinal nerve blocks in the lower abdomen for the pain of inguinal hernia repair, rectus sheath blocks in the anterior abdominal wall for umbilical hernia repair, and axillary nerve block for surgery of the forearm, elbow, or hand. In the past, anesthesiologists performed peripheral nerve blockade by observing body landmarks and manually feeling where the needle was placed as it penetrated the anterior abdominal wall. Now, when ultrasound is used in combination with these techniques, it provides a greater degree of accuracy and may also improve the safety of this type of nerve blockade.

Anesthesiologists are using ultrasonography more and more as a guide to nerve blockade in both adults and children. Because children typically undergo general anesthesia before nerve blocks, they are unable to communicate any procedure-related pain that they might experience if awake. Ultrasonography allows anesthesiologists to see the needle, nerves, and surrounding structures during the block procedure, which potentially adds an important measure of safety to pediatric anesthesia.

Ultrasound guidance for blocks within the adult spine, particularly spinals and epidurals, is somewhat limited by the fully developed bony structures. In contrast, a child's low body fat and reduced bone mineralization allows better ultrasound penetration and produces more useful spinal images. For this reason, ultrasound guidance has become more popular among anesthesiologists for the placement of neuraxial blocks in children than in adults. The rectus sheath block performed in the anterior abdomen is another nerve block that lends itself to ultrasound guidance. The combination of the anesthesiologist's observations and his or her palpation of body landmarks, plus ultrasound imaging, may improve the safety of rectus sheath blocks by keeping the needle from penetrating into the abdominal cavity.

Pregnancy and Childbirth

Obstetrics is a specialized area of anesthesia care. A woman and fetus compose a single biological system but are two individual patients, both of whom must be considered when medical therapy is provided. Furthermore, labor and delivery are natural physiological processes—the culmination of nine months of fetal growth and development—in contrast to surgical procedures, which are used to treat disease and disorder. The ideal birth situation is when a woman labors without drugs or medical interventions, since any drug could potentially cause an adverse or allergic response that could affect both her and the fetus. In reality, many women have severe or intolerable pain during labor and delivery, and anesthesia can positively affect both the safety and the humanity of the birth process.

As noted in chapter 2, general anesthesia was once commonly used during childbirth. Physicians used chloroform and ether to make women insensible or unconscious during labor well into the twentieth century. The clear disadvantages of general anesthesia in obstetric care have since become apparent. Because of the accumulation of fatty tissue, the increasing size of the breasts, and the swelling (especially in the inner aspect of the throat) of a pregnant woman's body, her airway becomes less accessible and difficult to manage during anesthesia. Failure to place a breathing tube, or to guarantee ongoing ventilation during general anesthesia, can threaten the life of both mother and fetus. In addition, a woman's stomach does not empty normally in the latter months of pregnancy, and if she undergoes general anesthesia, she is at risk of regurgitating toxic acidic stomach contents into her airway and lungs (a potentially fatal complication). For this reason, if general anesthesia is necessary for delivery, clinicians place great emphasis on securing the airway with a cuffed tube in the trachea to guard against regurgitation, which can be quite challenging given the anatomic changes noted above.

Another potential danger of general anesthesia in obstetric care is that it requires the use of six to eight different medications to produce deep unconsciousness and muscle relaxation in a patient. How well these drugs work depends on their ability to cross the natural protective barrier between the blood and the brain, which is typically a desirable characteristic of anesthetic drugs. Unfortunately, in the pregnant woman, this characteristic also allows anesthetic medications to cross the placenta and affect the fetus. A newborn who has been affected by anesthetic drugs may be sedated when delivered, requiring vigorous stimulation, oxygen, or even life-support equipment. For all these reasons, general anesthesia is undesirable during the birth process, if it can be safely avoided.

On the other hand, regional anesthesia has many advantages in obstetrical care and has become the preferred way to manage the pain of labor and delivery. There are obvious psychosocial benefits of regional anesthesia during the birth process. The woman is able to remain alert and participate in the delivery. The moment the child is delivered, she can hear its first cry. Within minutes, she is able to see and caress her vigorous newborn. Bonding begins immediately. Because the adverse effects of general anesthesia are avoided, the quality of this very human experience is greatly enhanced. In addition, the new father can accompany the laboring mother during the delivery process, encouraging her and even participating in the delivery. Regional techniques allow active participation in the arrival of a new baby.

Before the widespread acceptance and availability of epidural blocks for labor and delivery, physicians frequently administered pain medication as intramuscular or intravenous injections to a laboring woman. They typically injected opioids, which can produce sedation and nausea in the mother and may cross the placenta to affect the fetus. Today, these medications are less frequently used or are used only in small quantities, especially in hospitals with active obstetric anesthesia services.

The process of labor can be divided into three stages: stage one begins with the onset of regular uterine contractions and ends when the *cervix*, the muscular passageway at the base of the uterus, becomes completely dilated. Stage two then commences—the phase in which the woman pushes to deliver the baby. During stage three, the placenta is delivered.

In the first phase of labor, women experience considerable pain from the waves of contractions that dilate the cervix, often referred to as *labor pain*. Anesthesiologists can effectively control this pain by administering medications through an epidural catheter. These epidural infusions of local anesthetics are of relatively low dosage, allowing effective relief of pain, yet maintaining a woman's strength in the legs and pelvis to allow pushing during the second stage of labor. Obstetricians generally call for an epidural to be placed when a woman's cervix is several centimeters dilated already. Although there is concern that epidural blocks initiated very early in labor may slow the birth process, recent evidence appears to refute this. In addition, researchers have found that epidurals do not appear to cause an increase in the rate of cesarean section or instrument delivery. Most modern service-oriented obstetric departments permit pregnant women to receive an epidural for pain control during labor if they so desire. If labor is prolonged because of the use of epidural infusions, this effect is not significant, and many other factors affect the high rates of cesarean section in the United States.

Epidurals offer several other advantages in addition to psychosocial benefits when used for labor pain. Foremost, they are renewable, or continuous. Anesthesiologists can use epidural catheters to infuse local anesthetics for as long as labor continues. Such infusions can also be tailored to the woman's discomfort. If there is inadequate pain relief, the infusion can be increased to meet the woman's needs. If the drug effect is too strong, and the woman has significant leg weakness that reduces her ability to move in the bed or to push, the infusion can be briefly stopped, or its rate can be reduced. Under these circumstances, the anesthesiologist could also choose to reduce the concentration of local anesthetic and to add low doses of opioid medications for pain relief with less nerve blockade (and thus less leg weakness). High opioid doses can cause nausea, respiratory depression, and itching, but low doses of opioids and local anesthetic can complement each other and help avoid these side effects. In many obstetric centers, women are given some degree of control over the amount of pain medication infused into the epidural space, allowing them to adjust for their own comfort. This is called *patient-controlled epidural anesthesia*, or PCEA.

Epidurals also provide certain favorable effects during labor and delivery that are not related to pain control. The dilation of blood vessels that accompanies epidural anesthesia affects uterine arteries and can improve uterine blood flow. This is particularly useful in pregnant women with *pre-eclampsia*, a disorder in which the woman develops high blood pressure, protein in the urine, and swelling of the extremities. In pre-eclampsia, blood vessel constriction in the uterus can limit blood flow. Epidurals also reduce high levels of biological substances in the bloodstream called *catecholamines*, which may cause uterine blood vessel constriction. These positive effects of epidurals on uterine blood flow in turn reduce adverse effects on the fetus.

Epidural blocks can be vital to obstetrical care in other ways as well. It is not uncommon for the umbilical cord to be compressed during labor, causing a drop in blood flow in the fetus. On special obstetric monitors, this drop in blood flow appears as a decrease in the fetal heart rate, called *fetal deceleration*, for an extended period after each uterine contraction. If this process is not responsive to physician maneuvers, such as changing the fetal position and administering oxygen and fluids, then the fetus must be delivered urgently with a cesarean section. Under these conditions, the anesthesiologist can quickly initiate a dense regional block that will control pain and allow the surgeon to make a painless surgical incision through the abdominal wall and uterus. Although a general anesthetic can be used in this setting, it is undesirable for the reasons stated previously. If an epidural catheter has already been placed for control of labor pain, then a rapid, profound regional block can be administered using the catheter, making a cesarean delivery possible with the greatest possible safety for both the fetus and the mother. In essence, the epidural can serve as a spinal block when a rapidly acting medication is used. Injection of a higher concentration of local anesthetic through the epidural catheter (as opposed to the relatively dilute solutions used for the pain of labor) will provide surgical anesthesia within just a few minutes.

Some women choose to have *tubal ligation* (tying of the fallopian tubes) immediately after the birth of their last planned baby. For these women, after the baby is delivered, an epidural that has been used for the pain of labor or cesarean section may also be used to provide anesthesia for the tubal ligation. The anesthesiologist can once again numb the abdomen to the desired level using the same epidural catheter. This re-use of an existing epidural allows women to avoid the risks and side effects of general anesthesia.

Spinal blocks are also commonly used in obstetric anesthesia. When cesarean section is a planned event rather than an urgent one, anesthesiologists usually use spinal blocks unless there is a reason to avoid this technique (such as a bleeding abnormality). Again, the prime advantage of spinal anesthesia is to avoid general anesthesia, which is favorable for both the baby and the mother. For a woman to be comfortable during cesarean section, she must be numb approximately to the level of her lower rib cage or breasts, which may make some women feel as if they are having difficulty breathing—though with reassurance from the medical team, this sensation is usually tolerable. It subsides over time.

Spinal anesthesia can also be used at the time of vaginal delivery when an epidural has not been placed. Termed a *saddle block*, this type of anesthesia is delivered in such a way as to numb only the saddle area, or *perineum*. Saddle blocks are less popular than they once were, because the numbness of the groin region also produces weakness of the pelvic muscles, making it difficult for the woman to effectively push the fetus out.

Anesthesiologists can also use a combined spinal-epidural block to control pain during delivery. In this procedure, the anesthesiologist initially inserts an epidural needle into the epidural space of the spine, and then pushes a very long spinal needle through the larger epidural needle until its tip extends beyond the end of the epidural needle and into the dural sac. When spinal fluid is visible from the needle, confirming that it has been placed in the spinal sac, the anesthesiologist injects a small dose of opioid medication (such as fentanyl) and sometimes a small dose of local anesthetic as well. The spinal needle is then removed and a catheter is threaded through the epidural needle into the epidural space. Anesthesiologists do not place medication into this catheter initially; all pain relief comes from the spinal injection of the opioid medication. The initial pain relief generally lasts for several hours of labor and causes minimal leg weakness, allowing the woman more freedom to move around.

When the opioid drug begins to wear off, and contractions again become painful, the anesthesiologist activates the epidural catheter with an infusion of local anesthetic medication (with or without additional opioid) to control pain during the remainder of labor. This combined technique is especially favorable for women who have previously delivered children and may come to the hospital already in advanced labor, requiring immediate pain relief. Short-lived, rapid-onset pain relief from the spinal opioid block for these women is ideal because they often deliver much more quickly than first-time mothers. If labor becomes prolonged in such circumstances, the anesthesiologist can begin the epidural infusion as part of the combined spinal-epidural block.

Anesthesiologists prefer regional anesthesia to general anesthesia in obstetrics. The opportunity for a woman to be alert throughout the birth process is perhaps the most obvious benefit, but safety considerations are the prime advantages of regional techniques in this setting. Both epidural and spinal blocks have much to offer in the obstetric setting, and the considerable risks of general anesthesia should be avoided whenever possible.

Obstructive Sleep Apnea

For patients who have a breathing disorder called *obstructive sleep apnea* (OSA), the benefits of regional anesthesia may be even greater than those for the general population. Patients with OSA are frequently, though not always, overweight and have a disturbed sleep pattern: many times each night, they briefly stop breathing for several seconds. The obstruction may be from redundant tissue in the airway, or may simply be a consequence of the patient's internal anatomy. In addition to having obstructed breathing at night, many of these patients also have a central disorder of respiration in which muscle tone drops and tissues begin to obstruct the airway during inhalation. This means that their central nervous system does not control respiration effectively when they sleep, and even without physical obstruction, they may not breathe at the proper rate or depth.

General anesthesia is a more pronounced risk for people with OSA than for the average person. With sedation alone, even before general anesthesia is induced, such people may develop severe obstruction to breathing, or may stop breathing altogether. Anesthesiologists must be very careful to avoid levels of sleepiness that might lead to breathing irregularities when sedating people who have this condition. If clinicians are not ready to immediately place a tracheal tube, the patient could be in serious danger.

People who have OSA are predisposed to breathing difficulties during anesthesia because they are sensitive to any sedating medications and to the muscle relaxation that frequently accompanies anesthesia; this relaxation allows pharyngeal tissues and the tongue to obstruct the airway to an even greater degree. Waking up from anesthesia is particularly difficult for patients with OSA, which makes the end of the surgical procedure riskier than usual. Even in the recovery room, such patients may lapse back into a state of poor ventilation or obstruction of the airway from residual anesthetic effects, sometimes making it necessary to place an emergency airway.

One of the most severe adversities that patients who have OSA face is their need for postoperative treatment of pain with opioid medications.

Although some minor surgical procedures result in pain that is manageable with postoperative acetaminophen (Tylenol) or anti-inflammatory agents such as ibuprofen, most surgeries that involve a significant incision or deep tissue dissection require stronger medication for pain. Opioids are the standard therapy, but they are respiratory depressants and pose a real risk for patients who have OSA.

Recent recognition of the unique risks faced by these patients, as well as a marked increase in the number of people who have OSA, has led the American Society of Anesthesiologists to develop guidelines to ensure the best and safest possible care of these patients. One of their important recommendations is use of regional anesthesia, such as a spinal anesthetic or a peripheral nerve block, instead of general anesthesia whenever possible. Another essential guideline is to reduce or eliminate the use of opioids in the management of postoperative pain; doing so effectively usually involves nerve blocks, and perhaps even continuous (catheter) nerve blocks for several days after surgery. Thus, regional anesthesia is a key component of ensuring perioperative safety of patients who have OSA.

Elderly People

Anesthesiologists encounter many surgical patients in their eighties and nineties who have cardiovascular disease, pulmonary disease, or dementia. Regional anesthesia techniques may be useful with these patients because they help avoid intubation and mechanical ventilation during surgery, both of which are stresses to the lungs and the heart. In addition, with peripheral nerve blockade, there is less likelihood of patients developing low blood pressure—a complication often seen with general anesthesia, or even with spinal and epidural blocks. Keeping blood pressure stable can be particularly beneficial in patients who have vascular disease that affects the heart or brain. Reducing the stress-related chemicals that are released by the body after surgery may also benefit such patients. These chemicals may disturb the function of many organs and even lead to progression of blood vessel blockages related to underlying atherosclerosis, with resultant heart attack or stroke.

Evidence supporting the use of regional anesthesia instead of general anesthesia in the elderly is not definitive. Researchers have found favorable results after the use of regional anesthesia (primarily spinal and epidural blocks) for *some* surgeries that are typically performed in elderly patients, such as prostate removal, cancer surgeries, and total joint replacements.

Although more definitive studies are needed before firm conclusions can be drawn, many anesthesiologists prefer to use regional techniques in elderly patients who have severe coexisting diseases because of the reduced disturbance of consciousness and heart and lung function, as well as better pain control.

❋ As physicians treat increasing numbers of elderly patients with dementia, they must also consider the effect of anesthetic medications on the brain cell function of these patients. Family members of patients with dementia often warn physicians that their loved ones simply cannot tolerate the sedatives or pain medications used in the postoperative period because these drugs may result in a severe deterioration of mental function. Recent data do suggest worsened dementia after general anesthesia, but it is not clear if regional anesthesia techniques preserve brain function. Researchers have recently established that postoperative pain, morphine use, and nausea are significantly reduced when regional anesthesia is used for hip fracture repair (a common operation for elderly patients) instead of general anesthesia. This finding may greatly benefit patients with dementia who become more confused by the administration of opioid pain medications, and it can be seen as an encouraging endorsement of what many anesthesiologists have already been practicing in this population for many years.

Chapter 10

Pain Therapy

 How is pain defined?

What are the different types of pain?

How does the nervous system receive and process painful stimuli?

How is pain measured?

How can physicians treat acute pain after surgery?

What are the advantages of a *multimodal* approach to pain management?

Does early treatment of surgical pain reduce the likelihood of chronic pain at the surgery site?

How is an effective pain management service run in a hospital or practice?

What can be done if pain management is inadequate?

Much of this book has dealt with the unpleasant sensation of pain during surgery and the postoperative period. While the thrust has been to highlight regional anesthesia techniques and how they complement other forms of anesthesia, other modalities can be called into play to manage acute postoperative pain. In this chapter, I discuss the specific nature of pain, how pain is processed by the body, and the many means by which physicians can alleviate pain.

The American Society of Regional Anesthesia and Pain Medicine (ASRA) defines pain as "an unpleasant stimulus which evokes an unpleasant reaction in the recipient." This definition provides an important insight: physicians treating pain must consider both the perception of the individual and the measurable effects produced by the pain stimulus. In other words, pain has both subjective and objective components.

There are several types of pain, including *somatic* pain, *visceral* pain, and *neuropathic* pain. The nerve fiber endings of the skin, joints, bones, and body wall (chest, abdomen, back) are sensitive and distinct in how they perceive stimuli. They identify painful stimuli quickly, causing a sharp and immediately uncomfortable sensation called *somatic* pain. When organs inside the body, such as the bowel or the liver, are injured or inflamed, a person may experience pain that is dull and hard to locate, called *visceral* pain. Visceral pain may be felt in a location other than where the injury is located, and it may be unclear exactly where the person is hurting. This type of pain often comes on more gradually than somatic pain. At times, one type of pain may precede another; for example, in appendicitis, discomfort typically begins with visceral pain in the abdomen and later changes to somatic pain in the right lower abdomen as the inflammation spreads outside the appendix to the body wall. A third type of pain, called *neuropathic* pain, is the result of injury to nerves themselves. Neuropathic pain often becomes chronic, lasting longer than the stimulus that caused the injury.

Many different types of stimuli produce pain, including cuts, blunt trauma, crush injuries, swelling, extreme temperatures, and chemical injuries. The skin and other tissues have specialized nerve endings that perceive these painful stimuli. When these nerve endings are excited, the sensory nerves carry electrical impulses back to the central nervous system via *axons* (the long nerve fibers that originate in the dorsal root ganglion near the spinal cord). Impulses travel from the source of the stimulus along the axons in the peripheral nerves and into the spinal cord, where they are processed and modified in the *dorsal horn* area at each level of the spinal cord. When this collection of nerve cells receives the stimuli, it sends them up the spinal cord (via collections of axons termed *tracts*) to special sensory areas of the brain. These sensory areas project the stimuli to emotional and recognition centers of the *cortex*, which is the thinking part of the brain. When stimuli reach the cortex, an individual becomes consciously aware of the sensation and can decide to act. In addition to this conscious perception of pain, the brain projects impulses back down to the spinal cord and to each level of perception, regulating the degree to which pain is sensed and transmitted. Numerous chemical messengers, called *neurotransmitters*, are active in this process.

Pain may be *acute* (pain that has a sudden onset and that is short lasting but severe) or *chronic* (pain that has a gradual onset and that persists). Most people who have surgery experience acute pain at the site of the incision, which fades away as healing occurs. In some individuals, however, acute pain from trauma can persist because of how the nervous system responds to injury and inflammation. This chronic pain can adversely affect a person's quality of life in many ways. Effective early management of postoperative pain, particularly by intercepting pain messages using local anesthetics in nerve blocks, appears to make it less likely that a person will develop chronic pain from surgical incisions.

Pain is difficult to measure because it is a sensation and is therefore subjective. In hospitals, most clinicians ask patients to describe their pain on a 0 to 10 scale. Pain less than 4 is mild—bothersome but not intolerable, and usually managed with oral analgesic medications. Pain in the range of 5 to 7 is considered moderate and may not respond as readily to oral medications. Multiple oral medications, intravenous (IV) opioids, or a combination of different treatment methods (called *modalities*) may be necessary to treat this level of pain. Pain levels higher than 7 are considered severe, requiring rapid treatment with potent IV opioids and often other modalities.

Pain after surgery usually responds well to opioids, local anesthetic blocks, or a combination of the two. Sometimes, pain may be mild or nonexistent as long as a patient is resting, but it may become severe when the affected area is moved. For example, coughing after chest or abdominal surgery can be excruciating, and moving a leg after total knee replacement can be so severe that patients refuse to move. After an orthopedic surgery, a patient's immobility interferes with physical therapy and rehabilitation. In extreme circumstances, lack of movement can lead to scarring, fibrosis, a "frozen" joint, and chronic dysfunction. For these reasons, effectively managing postoperative pain is important for the long-term health of the patient.

Acute pain related to surgery can be managed in various ways, including the use of several classes of medications with specific actions on the nervous system. The pharmacological approach to managing pain has become increasingly sophisticated as pain specialists have learned more about the complex mechanisms behind how the human body registers, processes, amplifies, and suppresses pain stimuli.

Because each class of medication has its potential toxicities and side effects, physicians often use multiple therapeutic agents simultaneously—a type of treatment called *multimodal* analgesia. Types of pain medication for managing acute pain include:

- opioids (e.g., morphine);
- anti-inflammatory drugs (e.g., ibuprofen [Motrin] and celecoxib [Celebrex]);
- gabapentin, which modifies the central nervous system response to pain; and
- N-methyl d-aspartate (NMDA) receptor antagonists, which act on spinal cord receptors to influence how pain is processed.

Multimodal analgesia also incorporates regional anesthesia techniques (neuraxial nerve blocks or peripheral nerve blocks) and, at times, wound infiltration with local anesthetic solutions. This approach allows anesthesiologists to use multiple interventions that complement each other and also better control the side effects of each intervention.

Local anesthetic medications are an indispensable part of the multimodal management of pain, especially during the perioperative period. Anesthesiologists commonly use these drugs with nerve blocks, and surgeons often inject local anesthetics into a patient's surgical incision. A new technique for alleviating surgical pain is to place a catheter within the surgical wound itself. Such catheters permit surgeons to direct a constant infusion of local anesthetic solution that reduces sensation by blocking the tiny nerve fibers at the surgery site. Wound infusion catheters are useful for large, painful incisions, such as those required for abdominal or pelvic exploration, but are less useful for small incisions used in minimally invasive surgery. It is unknown whether the pain relief provided by this type of infusion is as effective as that of an epidural or peripheral nerve block catheter, but it appears to be at least as effective as IV morphine, if not more so, and can shorten and improve the quality of recovery time after major surgery.

In addition to nerve blocks and pain medications, physical measures may be employed to control pain. The inflammatory response after surgery is intense and can be modified by cooling techniques, so, for example, some clinicians use ice or cold water to provide a degree of numbness, at least to the surface tissues, and to control swelling and inflammation. Swelling, a component of inflammation and a consequence of holding a limb in one position, is an unpleasant sensation. Ice, elevation, and some gentle motion (when permitted) all help control swelling. Although these physical measures might not alleviate pain entirely, they offer an extra bit of comfort that allows patients to relax and concentrate on something other than pain during the early postoperative period.

Additional physical measures that physicians and other health care providers may use to make patients more comfortable after surgery include magnets, massage, acupuncture, and electrical nerve stimulation through the skin. Of these, acupuncture has shown the most promise. Acupuncturists insert tiny needles into the skin at pre-established points to influence how the body recognizes and processes pain. In some studies, acupuncture is almost as effective as mild oral analgesics in controlling pain. Unfortunately, most clinicians do not incorporate such physical measures (except the use of ice or cold water) consistently into postoperative pain-control regimens.

The timing of pain intervention is important. When patients are scheduled for surgery, anesthesiologists can begin treating them even before they experience any pain. The idea behind this pre-emptive pain relief is that blocking pain before it begins more effectively suppresses pain than trying to control it after it is established. Although there is a lack of solid scientific evidence supporting this idea, many anesthesiologists believe that pain control is more effective if it begins before surgery. Thus, anesthesiologists usually administer IV opioid drugs before anesthesia is begun, and they perform nerve blocks (if part of the anesthetic plan) before surgery. Other examples of pre-emptive and continuous analgesia for surgery include infusion of local anesthetics through an epidural catheter and administration of nonsteroidal anti-inflammatory medications, acetaminophen, or other analgesic drugs.

Integrating all the components of pain management can be logistically challenging. It is relatively simple to write orders for pain medications or write prescriptions for oral medications to be taken at home. On the other hand, pulling together a multimodal approach—standard preoperative medications, certain drugs provided consistently during the operation itself, and postoperative pain regimens that incorporate drugs that act at multiple sites—requires a major commitment from surgeons, anesthesiologists, and staff. Physicians must organize standardized regimens, or *pathways*, and then educate the staff to effectively use these pathways.

Even more time consuming, and certainly more complex, is the delivery of regional anesthetic blocks as a routine part of the pain-control regimen. To allow anesthesiologists time to perform nerve blocks without delaying surgery, patients must arrive early to the preoperative area, must be prescreened for major medical conditions that might affect anesthesia interventions, and must have a signed and up-to-date surgical consent form. Placing a nerve block requires

- a certain amount of time for placement;
- dedicated space, personnel, and equipment;
- sedation drugs;
- an ample supply of local anesthetics and nerve block-specific equipment (such as nerve stimulators and ultrasound machines); and
- various accessories, such as gel, skin preparation solution, syringes, towels, and gloves.

Placing *catheters* for continuous nerve blockade involves more of everything: time, effort, equipment, money, and patience. Not all anesthesia practices are able to provide these items and therefore are not consistently able to offer peripheral nerve block services.

Before deciding to integrate routine regional anesthetic blocks for patients in a busy anesthesia practice, physicians must consider how providing this service will affect their practice in terms of both administration and finances. Educational programs must be created for the surgeons, the perioperative nurses, and the anesthesiologists themselves, and additional staff may be required. Despite these challenges, there is definitely a national trend toward providing more regional anesthesia in practices today. The emphasis in anesthesia has shifted from only ensuring safe operative care to playing a greater role in postoperative care of the surgical patient.

After a patient's immediate recovery from surgery, anesthesiologists continue to manage his or her pain in various ways, depending on whether the patient is going home on the day of surgery. For outpatient surgery, pain is usually controlled through oral medications prescribed by the surgeon. At some hospitals or surgery centers, it is possible to have prescriptions filled at an on-site pharmacy, so patients can take the pain medications home when they are discharged. Otherwise, the patient may need to send a friend or family member to fill the prescriptions. If a nerve block has been placed, it will provide significant pain relief until it resolves.

Single-shot blocks usually last 8 to 24 hours, depending on the medication used and the patient's unique tissue characteristics. Ideally, a nerve block will provide a period of relief that allows a patient to get a good night's sleep on the day of surgery; however, blocks often wear off late in the evening or in the middle of the night after surgery. In my practice, I counsel patients to begin taking oral pain medications even before pain begins, which helps them transition from the block to oral analgesics for pain control.

For inpatient surgery, which is usually more extensive than outpatient surgery, pain is likely to be more severe. Anesthesiologists or surgeons will continue administering IV opioids for one to three days after patients leave the post-anesthesia care unit (PACU). The opioids may be administered with a patient-controlled analgesia (PCA) pump or by periodic injections. The surgeon usually directs this type of care by writing postoperative orders, but an *acute pain team* of anesthesiology providers may be involved. Once again, even if nerve blocks are performed, analgesic drugs will be available to help the patient transition to medications for managing pain and to cover any pain not effectively treated by the local anesthetics.

If physicians expect pain to be prolonged in a patient, as it may be with extensive orthopedic procedures or major abdominal surgery, they often choose to use a continuous form of regional anesthesia. Anesthesiologists deliver this type of anesthesia via a catheter in the spine (an epidural) or via a peripheral nerve block catheter (figure 10.1). Peripheral nerve block catheters, which are increasingly being used for outpatient procedures, provide pain relief for several days even when the patient returns home. After a specified time, the catheter is removed and discarded; pumps may also be discarded or may need to be returned to the hospital. Recent evidence suggests that ultrasound guidance allows more efficient and possibly more accurate placement of these catheters. The continuous pumps used with peripheral nerve block catheters are usually automatic, reliably delivering local anesthetic solution without input from the patient. Many devices also allow the patient to provide an extra measure of local anesthetic by pushing a button, which is similar to the familiar PCA pumps.

Considering how many factors must be addressed to provide effective pain relief for a patient who has undergone surgery, it is not surprising that things do not always go as planned. Adequate pain management requires attentive physicians, responsive nurses, effective medications delivered at the appropriate time, nerve blocks and catheters that function

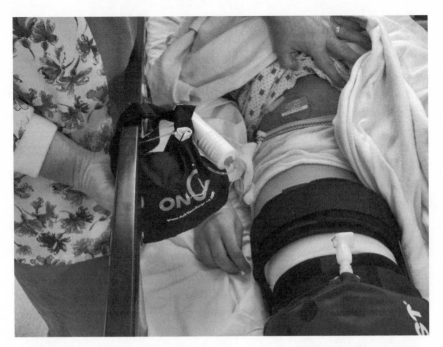

Figure 10.1 This patient has undergone knee surgery. Before surgery, a femoral nerve block was placed in the upper front of the thigh to control postoperative pain. Because the pain of this ligament reconstruction, which involved anchoring into bone, is expected to last several days, a catheter (tiny, hollow, flexible tube) was inserted through the nerve block needle and left in place. It allows a small disposable pump to infuse a dilute local anesthetic solution to the area around the nerve for the next three days, optimizing pain control and permitting improved joint mobility for passive range-of-motion exercises.

properly, and an accurate prediction by the anesthesiologist about which nerves will be affected during surgery. If any of these elements is deficient, the patient may experience pain.

What happens if you don't have adequate pain relief? Who will help you? The answer depends on your surgeon, hospital, and anesthesiology group, and the organization of their services, which can vary considerably. If you did not have a nerve block, your surgeon is usually responsible for writing prescriptions before you go home, or, for inpatients, for providing the nurses with orders for pain therapy. If you did undergo a nerve block or if you have a nerve block catheter, a member of the anesthesiology service will usually contact you by phone at your home on the day after surgery, or will visit you if you are in the hospital, to assess and modify your pain management. If you are receiving a continuous nerve block through a catheter, the anesthesiology service will generally contact you periodically until the catheter is removed; after that, the responsibility for pain control usually reverts to the surgeon.

If your pain becomes severe despite the therapy provided after surgery, you should contact the proper physician (your surgeon or anesthesiologist). If you are at home, make a phone call to the surgeon's office or to the anesthesiologist on-call; he or she may be able to modify your pain control regimen. The physician may change your prescribed medications, increase the dosage, counsel you about proper use of the catheter device, suggest a change in your body position, or (in the extreme) recommend that you visit the emergency department for an injection of pain medication. Rarely, after outpatient surgery, it may be necessary for a patient to return to the hospital for a repeated nerve block or replacement of a nerve block catheter that is not functioning optimally.

Patients who are admitted to the hospital after surgery usually have considerably less anxiety about managing their pain because they have a nurse close by at all times. The intensity of pain for such procedures is often greater, however, and just as pain may be an issue for outpatients, inpatient pain relief after surgery may also be inadequate. A request to the nurse should bring relief, either in the form of an additional dose of pain medication or a call to the surgical or anesthesia team to address the problem. Interventions may include an increase in the strength of oral pain medications, an increase in the dose of intravenous opioids, the addition of a new class of medications for pain, or the addition of new nerve blocks or catheters. Even simple interventions, such as loosening a brace or cast, increasing the frequency of ice bag placement (or replacing the cold water in the cuff), or changing the position of a limb can have dramatic effects on pain (figure 10.2).

Pain is an unavoidable consequence of surgical therapy. For many minor procedures, pain is easily managed with a prescription for oral opioid or anti-inflammatory medications. For major surgeries (inpatient or outpatient), pain will be more severe and may last longer. In any case, you should discuss the plan for pain management during the preoperative interview with your anesthesiologist. He or she has many different ways to control pain and ease your discomfort, including injecting potent opioid

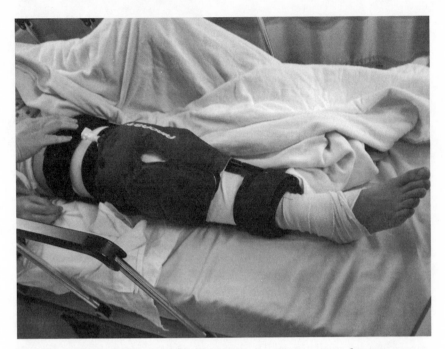

Figure 10.2 Elaborate braces are often placed on extremities after surgery, both to prevent motions that might be detrimental to the surgical repair in the early phases of healing and to provide protection. Motions of the limb are allowed greater range as healing progresses and repaired tissues gain strength. If not placed appropriately, or if applied too tightly, such immobilizing devices can result in inappropriate pressure on the extremity, with skin irritation or breakdown, or more detrimentally, nerve compromise.

medications or providing a patient-controlled pump, administering other drugs that take advantage of the multimodal approach to pain (such as anti-inflammatories), and using regional anesthesia (either as single injections or with continuous catheters).

I hope that after reading this book you are prepared to confidently discuss these techniques with members of your anesthesia team. Thinking about pain management before surgery and asking relevant questions during the preoperative interview will help you feel at ease when you consent to anesthesia and other methods of controlling pain.

References and Suggested Reading

Chapter 1. Introduction to Anesthesia and Surgery

American Board of Anesthesiology, www.theaba.org, accessed June 30, 2009.

American Society of Anesthesiologists. Practice Parameters. "Basic anesthesia monitoring standards 2005." www.asahq.org. Accessed June 6, 2009.

American Society of Anesthesiologists. Practice Parameters. "Continuum of depth of anesthesia—Definition of general anesthesia and levels of sedation/analgesia 2004." www.asahq.org. Accessed June 5, 2009.

American Society of Perianesthesia Nurses, www.aspan.org, accessed June 23, 2009.

Burkle CM, Sands RP, Bacon DR. "Beyond blocks: The history of the development of techniques in regional anesthesia," in: Raj PP (ed.) *Textbook of Regional Anesthesia.* New York: Churchill Livingstone, 2002. pp. 22–32.

Chung F, Mezei G. Factors contributing to a prolonged stay after ambulatory surgery. Anesth Analg 1999;89:1352–59.

Fleisher L. "Preoperative evaluation," in: Barash PG, Cullen BF, Stoelting RK (eds.) *Clinical Anesthesia,* 4th ed. Philadelphia: Lippincott, Williams, and Wilkins, 2001. pp. 473–90.

Hartrick CT. Multimodal postoperative pain management. Am J Health-Syst Pharm 2004;61:S4–S10.

Kohn LT, Corrigan JM, Donaldson MS (editors). *The Institute of Medicine: To Err Is Human.* Washington, D.C.: National Academy Press, 2001. pp. 164–65.

Lichtor L. "Anesthesia for ambulatory surgery," in: Barash PG, Cullen BF, Stoelting RK (eds.) *Clinical Anesthesia,* 4th ed. Philadelphia: Lippincott, Williams, and Wilkins, 2001. pp. 1217–38.

Tosky JA, Bacon DR, Calverley RK. "The history of anesthesiology," in: Barash PG, Cullen BF, Stoelting RK (eds.) *Clinical Anesthesia,* 4th ed. Philadelphia: Lippincott, Williams, and Wilkins, 2001. pp. 3–24.

Williams BA, Kentor ML, Vogt MT, Bogt WB, Coley KC, Williams JP, Roberts MS, Chelly JE, Harner CD, Fu FH. Economics of nerve block pain management after anterior cruciate ligament reconstruction. Anesthesiology 2004;100:697–706.

Chapter 2. A Brief History of Anesthesia

Burkle CM, Sands RP, Bacon DR. "Beyond blocks: The history of the development of techniques in regional anesthesia," in: Raj PP (ed.) *Textbook of Regional Anesthesia*. New York: Churchill Livingstone, 2002. pp. 22–32.
Fenster JM. *Ether Day: The Strange Tale of America's Greatest Medical Discovery and the Haunted Men Who Made It*. New York: Harper Collins, 2002.
Fradir DB. *We Have Conquered Pain: The Discovery of Anesthesia*. New York: Margaret K. McElderry Publishing (Simon and Schuster), 1996.
Kohn LT, Corrigan JM, Donaldson MS (editors). *The Institute of Medicine: To Err Is Human*. Washington, D.C.: National Academy Press, 2001. pp. 164–65.
Tosky JA, Bacon DR, Calverley RK. "The history of anesthesiology," in: Barash PG, Cullen BF, Stoelting RK (eds.) *Clinical Anesthesia*, 4th ed. Philadelphia: Lippincott, Williams, and Wilkins, 2001. pp. 3–24.

Chapter 3. General Anesthesia

Aldrete JA. The postanesthesia discharge score revisited. J Clin Anesth 1995;7:89–91.
American Society of Anesthesiologists. "Monitoring Standards." www.asahq.org. Accessed July 27, 2009.
Apfel CC, Korttila K, Abdalla M, et al. A factorial trial of six interventions for the prevention of postoperative nausea and vomiting. New Engl J Med 2004;350:2441–51.
Camu F. Side effects of opioids in postoperative pain treatment. Acta Anaesth Belgica 1996;47:105–109.
Chiu JW, White PF. "Nonopioid intravenous anesthesia," in: Barash PG, Cullen BF, Stoelting RK (eds.) *Clinical Anesthesia*, 4th ed. Philadelphia: Lippincott, Williams, and Wilkins, 2001. pp. 327–44.
Chung F. Recovery patterns and home-readiness after ambulatory surgery. Anesth Analg 1999;88:896–902.
Coda BA. "Opioids," in: Barash PG, Cullen BF, Stoelting RK (eds.) *Clinical Anesthesia*, 4th ed. Philadelphia: Lippincott, Williams, and Wilkins, 2001. pp. 345–76.
Eger II EI, Gong D, Koblin DD, et al. Effect of anesthetic duration on kinetic and recovery characteristics of desflurane versus sevoflurane (plus compound A) in volunteers. Anesth Analg 1998;86:414–21.
Gan TJ, Glass PS, Windsor A, et al. Bispectral index monitoring allows faster

emergence and improved recovery from propofol, alfenanil, and nitrous oxide anesthesia. Anesthesiology 1997;87:808–15.

Gan TJ, Sloan F, Dear G, et al. How much are patients willing to pay to avoid postoperative nausea and vomiting? Anesth Analg 2001;92:393–400.

Gupta A, Stierer T, Zuckerman R, et al. Comparison of recovery profile after ambulatory anesthesia with propofol, isoflurane, sevoflurane and desflurane: A systematic review. Anesth Analg 2004;98:632–41.

Higgins PP, Chung F, Mezei G. Postoperative sore throat after ambulatory surgery. Br J Anaesth 2002;88:582–84.

Joshi GP. Multimodal analgesia techniques of ambulatory surgery. Int Anesth Clin 2005;197–204.

Kehlet H, Dahl JB. The value of "multimodal" or "balanced analgesia" in postoperative pain treatment. Anesth Analg 1993;77:1048–56.

Kissin I. Depth of anesthesia and bispectral index monitoring. Anesth Analg 2000;90:1114–17.

O'Keefe ST, Chonchubhair AN. Postoperative delirium in the elderly. Br J Anaesth 1994;73:673–87.

Orebaugh SL. *Airway Management: Tools and Techniques.* Philadelphia: Lippincott, Williams, and Wilkins, 2006.

Pavlin DJ, Rapp SE, Polissar NL, et al. Factors affecting discharge times in adult outpatients. Anesth Analg 1998;87:816–26.

Scuderi PE, James R, Harris L, et al. Multimodal management prevents early postoperative vomiting after outpatient laparoscopy. Anesth Analg 2000;91:1246–52.

Tinker JH. Role of monitoring devices in prevention of anesthetic mishaps: A closed claims analysis. Anesthesiology 1989;71:535–40.

Verghese C, Brimacombe J. Survey of laryngeal mask airway usage in 119,110 patients—Safety and efficacy for conventional and nonconventional usage. Anaesthesia 1996;82:129–33.

White PF. Multimodal analgesia: Its role in preventing postoperative pain. Curr Opin Invest Drugs 2008;9:76–82.

Chapter 4. Complications, Risk Assessment, and Safety

Ahlers O, Nachtigall I, Lenze J, et al. Intraoperative thoracic epidural anaesthesia attenuates stress-induced immunosuppression in patients undergoing major abdominal surgery. Br J Anaesth 2008;101:781–87.

American Association of Nurse Anesthetists, www.aana.org, accessed June 7, 2009.

American College of Cardiology / American Heart Association Task Force on Practice Guidelines. ACC/AHA 2007 guidelines on perioperative cardiovascular evaluation and care for noncardiac surgery: Executive summary. Anesth Analg 2008;106:685–712.

American Society of Anesthesiologists' Task Force on the Management of the Difficult Airway. Practice guidelines for the management of the difficult airway. Anesthesiology 2003;98:1269–77.

Anesthesia Patient Safety Foundation, www.apsf.org, accessed June 6, 2009.

Benumof JL. Laryngeal mask airway and the ASA difficult airway algorithm. Anesthesiology 1996;84:686–99.

Benumof JL. Management of the difficult adult airway. With special emphasis on awake tracheal intubation. Anesthesiology 1991;75:1087–1110.

Chopra V, Plaisance B, Cavusoglu E, et al. Perioperative beta-blockers for major noncardiac surgery: Primum non nocere. Am J Med 2009;122:222–29.

Cucchiara RF, Black S. Corneal abrasion during anesthesia and surgery. Anesthesiology 1988;69:978–79.

Currie M, Kerridge RK, Bacon AK, Williamson JA. Crisis management during anaesthesia: Anaphylaxis and allergy. Quality and safety in health care. 2005;14:19.

Dzankic S, Pastor D, Gonzalez C, Leung JM. The prevalence and predictive value of abnormal preoperative laboratory tests in elderly surgical patients. Anesth Analg 2001;93:301–308.

Fleisher LA. "Preoperative evaluation," in: Barash PG, Cullen BF, Stoelting RK (eds.) Clinical Anesthesia, 4th ed. Philadelphia: Lippincott, Williams, and Wilkins, 2001. pp. 473–89.

Fleisher LA. Real-time intraoperative monitoring of myocardial ischemia in noncardiac surgery. Anesthesiology 2000;92:1183–88.

Fleisher LA. Risk indices: What is their value to the clinician and patient. Anesthesiology 2001;94:191–93.

Fleisher LA, Beckman JA, Brown KA, et al. ACC/AHA guideline update on perioperative cardiovascular evaluation for noncardiac surgery: Focused update on perioperative beta-blockade therapy. Anesth Analg 2007;104:15–26.

Kawashima Y, Takahashi S, Suzuki M, et al. Anesthesia-related mortality and morbidity over a 5 year period in 2,363,038 patients in Japan. Acta Anaesth Scand 2003;47:809–17.

Larach MG, Brandon BW, Allan G, Gronert GA, et al. Cardiac arrests and deaths associated with malignant hyperthermia in North America from 1987–2006. Anesthesiology 2008;108:603–11.

Loepke AW, Soriano SG. An assessment of the effects of general anesthetics on developing brain structure and cognitive function. Anesth Analg 2008; 1681–1707.

McFalls EO, Ward HB, Mortitz TE, et al. Coronary artery revascularization before elective major vascular surgery. N Engl J Med 2004;351:2795–2804.

Mertes PM, Laxenaire MC, Alla F. Anaphylactic and anaphylactoid reactions occurring during anesthesia in France in 1999–2000. Anesthesiology 2003;99:536–45.

Monk TG, Saini V, Weldon BC, Sigl JC. Anesthetic management and one-year mortality after noncardiac surgery. Anesth Analg 2005;100:4–10.

National Patient Safety Foundation, www.npsf.org, accessed June 6, 2009.

Newland MC, Ellis SJ, Lydiatt CA. Anesthetic-related cardiac arrest and its mortality. Anesthesiology 2002;97:108–15.

Newman NJ. Perioperative visual loss after nonocular surgeries. Am J Ophthalm 2008;145:604–10.

Newman S, Stygall J, Shashivadan H, et al. Postoperative cognitive dysfunction after noncardiac surgery. Anesthesiology 2007;106:572–90.

Niwa Y, Nakae A, Ogawa M, et al. Arytenoid dislocation after cardiac surgery. Acta Anaesth Scand 2007;51:1397–1400.

Orebaugh SL. *Airway Management: Tools and Techniques.* Philadelphia: Lippincott, Williams, and Wilkins, 2006.

Palda VA, Detsky AS. Perioperative assessment and management of risk from coronary artery disease. Ann Int Med 1997;127:313–28.

Pasternak LR. Preoperative laboratory testing: General issues and considerations. Anesth Clin North Am 2004;22:13–25.

POISE study group, Devereaux PJ, Yang H, Yusuf S, et al. Effects of extended-release metoprolol succinate in patients undergoing non-cardiac surgery (POISE trial): A randomized controlled trial. Lancet 2008;371:1839–47.

Sessler DI. Long-term consequences of anesthesia management. Anesthesiology 2009;111:1–4.

Smetana GW, Lawrence VA, Cornell JE. Preoperative pulmonary risk stratification for noncardiac surgery: Systematic review for the American College of Chest Physicians. Ann Int Med 2006;144:581–95.

Stambough JL, Dolan D, Werner R, Godfrey E. Ophthalmologic complications associated with the prone position during spine surgery. J Am Acad Ortho Surg 2007;11:156–65.

Warner MA, Warner ME, Weber JG. Clinical significance of pulmonary aspiration during the perioperative period. Anesthesiology 1993;78:56–66.

Chapter 5. Regional Anesthesia

American Society of Anesthesiologists, "Conduction anesthesia," www.asahq.org, accessed August 27, 2009.

American Society of Anesthesiologists, "Guidelines on obstructive sleep apnea," www.asahq.org, accessed August 27, 2009.

Ben-David B, Chelly JE. Continuous peripheral neural blockade for postoperative analgesia: Practical advantages. Anesth Analg 2003;2003;96:1537–39.

Bernards CM. "Epidural and Spinal Anesthesia," in: Barash PG, Cullen BF, Stoelting RK (eds.) *Clinical Anesthesia,* 4th ed. Philadelphia: Lippincott, Williams, and Wilkins, 2001. pp. 689–713.

Butterworth JF, Strichartz GR. The molecular mechanisms by which local anesthetics produce impulse blockade: A review. Anesthesiology 1990;72:711–34.

Casati A. "Local anesthetic solutions," in: Chelly JE (ed.) *Peripheral Nerve Blocks: A Color Atlas*, 3rd edition. Philadelphia: Wolters Kluwer/Lippincott, Williams, and Wilkins, 2009. pp. 12–19.

Chelly JE, et al. Continuous femoral blocks improve recovery and outcome of patients undergoing total knee arthroplasty. J Arthroplasty 2001;16:436–45.

Cheng GS, Choy LP, Ilfeld BM. Regional anesthesia at home. Curr Opin Anesthesiology 2008;21:488–93.

Dahl JB, Rosenburg J, Kehlet H. Effect of thoracic epidural etidocaine 1.5% on somatosensory evoked potentials, cortisol and glucose during cholecystectomy. Acta Anaesthesiol Scand 1992;36:378–82.

Eisenach JC. Treating and preventing chronic pain: A view from the spinal cord. Bonica Lecture. Reg Anesth Pain Med 2006;31:146–51.

Hadzic A, Kraca PE, Hobeika P, et al. Peripheral nerve blocks result in superior recovery profile compared with general anesthesia in outpatient knee arthroscopy. Anesth Analg 2005;100:976–81.

Hadzic A, Williams BA, Karaca PE, et al. For outpatient rotator cuff surgery, nerve block anesthesia provides superior same-day recovery over general anesthesia. Anesthesiology 2005;102:1001–1007.

Ilfeld B, Vandenborne K, Duncan PW, et al. Ambulatory continuous interscalene nerve blocks decrease the time to discharge readiness after total shoulder arthroplasty: A randomized, triple-masked, placebo-controlled study. Anesthesiology 2006;105:999–1007.

Ilfeld BM, Le LT, Meyer RS, Mariano ER, et al. Ambulatory continuous femoral nerve blocks decrease time to discharge readiness after tricompartment total knee arthroplasty: A randomized, triple-masked, placebo-controlled study. Anesthesiology 2008;703–13.

Isono S. Obstructive sleep apnea of obese adults. Anesthesiology 2009;110:908–21.

Kehlet H. Effects of postoperative pain management on outcome: Current status and future strategies. Arch Surg 2004;389:244–49.

Kehlet H, Jensen TS, Woolf CJ. Persistent postsurgical pain: Risk factors and prevention. Lancet 2006;367:1618–25.

Kidd BL, Urban LA. Mechanisms of inflammatory pain. Br J Anaesth 2001; 87:3–11.

Lee LA, Posner KL, Domino KB, et al. Injuries associated with regional anesthesia in the 1980s and 1990s. Anesthesiology 2004;101:143–52.

Liu S. Continuous peripheral nerve blockade and PCA for postoperative analgesia. Anest Analg 2006;102:248.

Liu S, Carpenter RL, Neal JM. Epidural anesthesia and analgesia: Their role in postoperative outcome. Anesthesiology 1995;82:1474–1506.

Liu SS. A comparison of regional versus general anesthesia for ambulatory anesthesia. Anesth Analg 2005;101:1634–42.

Liu SS, Carpenter RL, Mackey DC, et al. Effects of perioperative analgesic
technique on rate of recovery after colon surgery. Anesthesiology 1995;83:
757–65.

Lou L, Sabar R, Kaye AD. "Local anesthetics," in: Raj PP (ed.) *Textbook of Regional
Anesthesia*. New York: Churchill Livingstone, 2002. pp. 177–214.

Lubenow TR, Ivankovich AD, McCarthy RJ. "Management of acute postoperative
pain," in: Barash PG, Cullen BF, Stoelting RK (eds.) *Clinical Anesthesia*, 4th ed.
Philadelphia: Lippincott, Williams, and Wilkins, 2001. pp. 1403–34.

Marino J, Russo J, Kenny M, et al. Continuous lumbar plexus block for
postoperative pain control after total hip arthroplasty. J Bone Joint Surg Am
2009;91:29–37.

Ong CK, Lirk P, Seymour RA, Jenkins BJ. The efficacy of preemptive analgesia
for acute postoperative pain management: A meta-analysis. Anesth Analg
2005;100:757–73.

Reina MA, de Andres J, Lopez A. "Subarachnoid and epidural anesthesia," in: Raj
PP (ed.) *Textbook of Regional Anesthesia*. New York: Churchill Livingstone, 2002.
pp. 307–25.

Rodgers A, Walker N, Schug S, et al. Reduction of postoperative mortality
and morbidity with epidural or spinal anaesthesia: Results from overview of
randomized trials. Br Med J 2000;321:1–12.

Schrenk P, Bettelheim P, Woisetschlager R, et al. Metabolic responses after
laparoscopic or open hernia repair. Surg Endosc 1996;10:628–32.

Senturk M, Ozcan PE, Talu GK, et al. The effects of three different analgesia
techniques on long-term post-thoracotomy pain. Anesth Analg 2002;94:
11–15.

Stannard C, Booth S. "Anatomy and Physiology of Pain," in: *Pain*, 2nd edition.
Edinburgh: Elsevier, 2004. pp. 4–11.

Willams BA, Kentor ML, Vogt MT, et al. Economics of nerve block pain
management after anterior cruciate ligament reconstruction. Anesthesiology
2004;100:697–706.

Williams BA, Kentor ML, Vogt MT, et al. Reduction of verbal pain scores after
anterior cruciate ligament reconstruction with 2-day continuous femoral nerve
block. Anesthesiology 2006;104:315–27.

Wu CL. "Efficacy of neuraxial and peripheral nerve blocks in acute pain
management," in: Raj PP (ed.) *Textbook of Regional Anesthesia*. New York:
Churchill Livingstone, 2002. pp. 873–893.

Chapter 6. Spinal Anesthesia and Epidural Anesthesia

American Society of Anesthesiologists, "Practice guidelines for obstetric anesthesia,"
www.asahq.org, accessed April 1, 2011.

Bauer C, Hentz J-G, Ducrocq X, Nicolas M, Oswald-Mammosser M, Steib A,
Dupeyron J-P. Lung function after lobectomy: A randomized, double-blinded

trial comparing thoracic epidural ropivacaione/sufentanily and intravenous morphine for patient-controlled analgesia. Anesth Analg 2007;105:238–44.

Celleno D, Capogna G, Constantino P, Catalano P. An anatomic study of the effects of dural puncture with different spinal needles. Reg Anesth 1993; 218–21.

Drasner K. "Subarachnoid," in: Hahn MB, McQuillan PM, Sheplock GJ (eds.) *Regional Anesthesia*. St. Louis: Mosby, 1996. pp. 2221–30.

Hogan Q. "Epidural," in: Hahn MB, McQuillan PM, Sheplock GJ (eds.) *Regional Anesthesia*. St. Louis: Mosby, 1996. pp. 213–220.

Joshi GP, Bonnet F, Shah R, Wilkinson RC, Camu F, Fischer B, Neugebauer EAM, Rawal N, Schug SA, Simanski C, Kehlet H. A systematic review of randomized trials evaluating regional techniques for post-thoracotomy analgesia. Anesth Analg 2008;107:1026–40.

Lavan'homme P, De Kock M, Waterloos H. Intraoperative epidural analgesia combined with ketamine provides effective preventive analgesia in patients undergoing major digestive surgery. Anesthesiology 2005;103:813–20.

Obata H, Saito S, Fujita N, Fuse Y, Ishizaki K, Goto F. Epidural block with mepivacaine before surgery reduces long-term post-thoracotomy pain. Can J Anaesth 1999;46:1127–32.

Raj PP. "Conduction blocks," in: Raj PP (ed.) *Textbook of Regional Anesthesia*. New York: Churchill Livingstone, 2002. pp. 285–306.

Reina MA, de Andres J, Lopez A. "Subarachnoid and epidural anesthesia" in: Raj PP (ed.) *Textbook of Regional Anesthesia*. New York: Churchill Livingstone, 2002. pp. 307–324.

Rodgers A, Walker N, Schug S, et al. Reduction of postoperative mortality and morbidity with epidural or spinal anaesthesia: Results from overview of randomized trials. Br Med J 2000;321:1–12.

Santos AC, O'Gorman DA, Finster M. "Obstetric anesthesia," in: Barash PG, Cullen BF, Stoelting RK (eds.) *Clinical Anesthesia,* 4th ed. Philadelphia: Lippincott, Williams, and Wilkins, 2001. pp. 1141–70.

Senturk M, Ozcan PE, Talu GK, Kiyan E, Camci E, Ozyalcin S, Dilege S, Pembeci K. The effects of three different analgesia techniques on long-term post-thoracotomy pain. Anesth Analg 2992;94:11–15.

Weller JF, Wu CL. "Does intraoperative regional anesthesia decrease perioperative blood loss?" in: Fleisher LA (ed.) *Evidence-based Practice of Anesthesiology*. Philadelphia: Saunders, 2004. pp. 283–86.

Willams BA, Kentor ML, Vogt MT, et al. Economics of nerve block pain management after anterior cruciate ligament reconstruction. Anesthesiology 2004;100:697–706.

Williams BA, Kentor ML, Vogt MT, et al. Reduction of verbal pain scores after anterior cruciate ligament reconstruction with 2-day continuous femoral nerve block. Anesthesiology 2006;104:315–27.

Wlody D. "What is the optimum management of postdural puncture headache?" in: Fleisher LA (ed.) *Evidence-based Practice of Anesthesiology.* Philadelphia: Saunders, 2004. pp. 314–17.

Chapter 7. Peripheral Nerve Blocks

American Society of Regional Anesthesia and Pain Medicine. "Clinical guidelines: Anticoagulation in regional anesthesia," www.asra.com, accessed October 19, 2009.

Chelly JE, Greger J, Gebhard R, et al. Continuous femoral blocks improve recovery and outcomes of patients undergoing total knee arthroplasty. J Arthroplasty 2001;16:436–45.

Gray AT. Ultrasound-guided regional anesthesia. Anesthesiology 2006;104:368–73.

Greengrass R, Steele S, Moretti G, et al. "Peripheral Nerve Blocks," in: Raj PP (ed.) *Textbook of Regional Anesthesia.* Philadelphia: Churchill Livingstone, 2002. pp. 325–78.

Hadzic A, Arliss J, Kerimoglu B, et al. A comparison of infraclavicular nerve block versus general anesthesia for hand and wrist day-case surgeries. Anesthesiology 2004;101:127–32.

Hadzic A, Vloka JD. *Peripheral Nerve Blockade.* New York: McGraw-Hill, 2004. pp. 9–28.

Hadzic A, Williams BA, Karaca PE, et al. For outpatient rotator cuff surgery, nerve block anesthesia provides superior same-day recovery over general anesthesia. Anesthesiology 2005;102:1001–1007.

Hogan Q. Finding nerves is not simple. Reg Anesth Pain Med 2003;28:367–71.

Ilfeld BM, Wright TW, Enneking K, et al. Joint range of motion after total shoulder arthroplasty with and without a continuous interscalene block: A retrospective, case-control study. Reg Anesth Pain Med 2005;30:429–33.

Karaca P, Hadzic A, Yufa M, et al. Painful paresthesiae are infrequent during brachial plexus localization using low current peripheral nerve stimulation. Reg Anesth Pain Med 2003;28:380–83.

Liu SS, Hodgson PS. "Local anesthetics," in: Barash PG, Cullen BF, Stoelting RK (eds.) *Clinical Anesthesia,* 4th ed. Philadelphia: Lippincott, Williams, and Wilkins, 2001. pp. 449–69.

Liu SS, Strodtbeck W, Richman J, et al. A comparison of regional versus general anesthesia for ambulatory anesthesia: A meta-analysis of controlled trials. Anesth Analg 2005;101:1634–42.

Marhofer P, Chan VW. Ultrasound-guided regional anesthesia: Current concepts and future trends. Anesth Analg 2007;104:1265–69.

McCartney CJ, Brull R, Chan VW, et al. Early but no long-term benefit of regional compared with general anesthesia for ambulatory hand surgery. Anesthesiology 2004;101:461–67.

Moore KL, Dalley AF. *Clinically Oriented Anatomy*, 4th edition. Philadelphia: Lippincott, Williams, and Wilkins, 1999. pp. 38–52.

Raj PP, de Andres J, Grossi P, et al. "Aids to localization of peripheral nerves," in: Raj PP (ed.) *Textbook of Regional Anesthesia*. Philadelphia: Churchill Livingstone, 2002. pp. 251–84.

Richman J, Liu SS, Courpas G, et al. Does continuous peripheral nerve block provide superior pain control to opioids: A meta-analysis. Anesth Analg 2006;120:248–57.

Sites BD, Spence BC, Gallagher J, et al. Regional anesthesia meets ultrasound: A specialty in transition. Acta Anaesth Scand 2008;52:456–66.

Williams BA, Kentor ML, Vogt MT, et al. The economics of nerve block pain management after anterior cruciate ligament reconstruction: Significant hospital cost savings via associate PACU bypass and same-day discharge. Anesthesiology 2004;100:697–706.

Chapter 8. Complications of Regional Anesthesia

American Society of Regional Anesthesia and Pain Medicine, "Guidelines on anticoagulation and regional anesthesia," www.asra.org, accessed December 12, 2009.

Auroy Y, Benhamou D, Bargues L, Ecoffey C, Falissar B, Mercier F, Bouaziz H, Samii K. Major complications of regional anesthesia in France. Anesthesiology 2002;97:1274–80.

Benumof JL. Permanent loss of cervical spinal cord function associated with interscalene block under general anesthesia. Anesthesiology 2000;93:1541–44.

Borgeat A, Ekatodramis G, Kalberer F, Benz C. Acute and nonacute complications associated with interscalene block and shoulder surgery. Anesthesiology 2001;95:875–80.

Brull R and McCartney CJL. Neurological complications after regional anesthesia: Contemporary estimates of risk. Anesth Analg 2007;104:965–74.

Chan VWS, Perlas A, McCartney CJL, Brull R, Xu D, Abbas S. Ultrasound guidance improves success rate of axillary brachial plexus block. Can J Anaesth 2007;54:176–82.

Covino BG, Lambert DH. "Epidural and spinal anesthesia," in: Barash PG, Cullen BF, Stoelting RK (eds.) *Clinical Anesthesia*, 2nd ed. Philadelphia: Lippincott, Williams, and Wilkins, 1992. pp. 809–40.

Cuvillon P, Ripart J, Lalourcey L, Veyrat E, L-Hermite J, Boisson C, Thouabtia E, Eledjam JJ. The continuous femoral nerve block catheter for postoperative analgesia: Bacterial colonization, infectious rate and adverse effects. Anesth Analg 2001;93:1045–49.

Gerancher JC, Liu SS. "Complications of neuraxial anesthesia," in: Benumof JL, Saidman LJ (eds.) *Anesthesia and Perioperative Complications*. St. Louis: Mosby, 1999. pp. 50–65.

Hogan QH. Pathophysiology of peripheral nerve injury during regional anesthesia. Reg Anesth Pain Med 2008;33:435–41.

Horlocker TT, Heit JA. Low molecular weight heparin: Biochemistry, pharmacology, perioperative prophylaxis regimens and guidelines for regional anesthesia management. Anesth Analg 1997;85:874–85.

Liu SS, Zayas VM, Gordon MA, Beathe JC, Maalouf DB, Paroli L, Ligouri GA, Ortiz J, Buschiazzo V, Ngeow J, Shetty T, Ya Deau JT. A prospective, randomized controlled trial comparing ultrasound versus nerve stimulator guidance for interscalene block for ambulatory shoulder surgery for postoperative neurologic symptoms. Anesth Analg 2009;109:265–71.

Mather LE, Copeland SE, Ladd LA. Acute toxicity of local anesthetics: Underlying pharmacokinetic and pharmacodynamic concepts. Reg Anesth Pain Med 2005;30:553–67.

Mulroy MF. Systemic toxicity and cardiotoxicity from local anesthetics: Incidence and preventive measures. Reg Anesth Pain Med 2002;27:556–61.

Neal JM, Bernards CM, Hadzic A, Hebl JR, Hogan QH, Horlocker TT, Lee LA, Rathmell JP, Sorenson EJ, Suresh S, Wedel DJ. ASRA practice advisory on neurologic complications in regional anesthesia and pain medicine. Reg Anesth Pain Med 2008;404–15.

Rosenberg PH, Veering BT, Urmey WF. Maximum recommended doses of local anesthetics: A multifactorial concept. Reg Anesth Pain Med 2004;29: 564–75.

Rosenblatt MA, Abal M, Fischer G, Itzkovic CJ, Eisenkraft JB. Successful use of a 20% lipid emulsion to resuscitate a patient after a presumed bupivacaine-related cardiac arrest. Anesthesiology 2006;105:217–18.

Stan TC, Krantz MA, Solomon DL, Poulos JG, Chaouki K. The incidence of neurovascular complications following axillary brachial plexus block using a transarterial approach. Reg Anesth 1995;20:486–92.

Weinberg G. Lipid infusion resuscitation for local anesthetic toxicity. Anesthesiology 2007;105:7–8.

Chapter 9. Regional Anesthesia for Special Populations

Children

Ecoffey C. "Regional anesthesia in children," in: Raj PP (ed.) *Textbook of Regional Anesthesia*. New York: Churchill Livingstone, 2002. pp. 379–396.

Tobias JD. "Fundamentals of ultrasound-guided pediatric regional anesthesia," in: Bigeleisen PE (ed.) *Ultrasound-Guided Regional Anesthesia and Pain Medicine*. Philadelphia: Wolters Kluwer Health/Lippincott, Williams, and Wilkins, 2010. pp. 163–70.

Tsui BC, Pillay JJ. Evidence-based medicine: Assessment of ultrasound imaging for regional anesthesia in infants, children and adolescents. Reg Anesth Pain Med 2010;35 (Suppl 1):47–54.

Tsui BCH, Suresh S. Ultrasound imaging for regional anesthesia in infants, children and adolescents. Anesthesiology 2010;112:473–92.

Yaster M, Hardart RA. "Pediatric pain management," in: Raj PP (ed.) *Textbook of Regional Anesthesia*. New York: Churchill Livingstone, 2002. pp. 1009–1032.

Pregnancy and Childbirth

American College of Obstetricians and Gynecologists, Committee on Obstetric Practice. Analgesia and cesarean delivery rates. ACOG Committee Opinion No. 269. Washington, D.C.: ACOG, 2002.

American College of Obstetricians and Gynecologists, Committee on Obstetric Practice. Pain relief in labor. ACOG Committee Opinion No. 231. Washington, D.C.: ACOG, 2002.

American Society of Anesthesiologists Statement on Pain Relief During Labor. Obstetrical Anesthesia Committee, 1999; amended 2009, www.asahq.org, accessed May 17, 2010.

Beilin Y. "Anesthesia for Cesarean delivery: Regional or general?" in: Fleisher LA (ed.) *Evidence-Based Practice of Anesthesiology*. Philadelphia: Saunders, 2004. pp. 401–406.

Finster M, Ralston DH, Pedersen H. "Perinatal pharmacology," in: Shnider SM, Levinson G (eds.) *Anesthesia for Obstetrics*, 3rd ed. Baltimore: Williams and Wilkins, 1993. pp. 71–79.

Sharma SK, Alexander JM, Messick G, et al. Cesarean delivery: A randomized trial of epidural analgesia versus intravenous meperidine during labor in nulliparous women. Anesthesiology 2002;96:546–51.

Shnider SM, Levinson G, Cosmi EV. "Obstetric anesthesia and uterine blood flow," in: Shnider SM, Levinson G (eds.) *Anesthesia for Obstetrics*, 3rd ed. Baltimore: Williams and Wilkins, 1993. pp. 29–51.

Wang F, Shen X, Guo X, Peng Y, Gu X. Epidural analgesia in the latent phase of labor and the risk of cesarean delivery: A five-year randomized, controlled trial. Anesthesiology 2009;111:871–80.

Weiss BM, Alon E, McKay RSF. "Efficacy and outcome of regional anesthesia techniques in obstetrics," in: Raj PP (ed.) *Textbook of Regional Anesthesia*. New York: Churchill Livingstone, 2002. pp. 907–56.

Obstructive Sleep Apnea

Benumof JL. Obstructive sleep apnea in the adult obese patient: Implications for airway management. J Clin Anesth 2001;13:144–56.

Isono S. Obstructive sleep apnea of obese adults: Pathophysiology and perioperative airway management. Anesthesiology 2009;110:908–21.

Practice guidelines for the perioperative management of patients with obstructive sleep apnea. Anesthesiology 2006;104:1081–93.

Rock P, Passannante A, Dorman T. "What is the optimal intraoperative and postoperative management of the Obstructive Sleep Apnea Patient?" in: Fleisher

LA (ed.) *Evidence-Based Practice of Anesthesiology.* Philadelphia: Saunders, 2004. pp. 253–57.

Ulnick KM, Debo RF. Postoperative treatment of the patient with obstructive sleep apnea. Otolaryngol Head Neck Surg 2000;122:233–36.

Elderly People

Macfarlane AJ, Prasad GA, Chan VW, Brull R. Does regional anesthesia improve outcome after total hip arthroplasty? A systematic review. Br J Anaesth 2009;103:335–45.

Newman S, Stylgell J, Hirani S, Shaefi S, Maze M. Postoperative cognitive dysfunction after noncardiac surgery: A systematic review. Anesthesiology 2007;106:572–90.

Ramaiah R, Lam AM. Postoperative cognitive dysfunction in the elderly. Anesth Clinics 2009;27:485–96.

Chapter 10. Pain Therapy

Beaussier M, El'Ayoubi H, Schiffer E, et al. Continuous perperitoneal infusion of ropivacaine provides effective analgesia and accelerates recovery after colo-rectal surgery: A randomized, double-blind, placebo-controlled study. Anesthesiology 2007;107:461–68.

Boezaart AP. Perineural infusion of local anesthetics. Anesthesiology 2006;104:872–80.

Buvanendran A, Kroin JS. Multimodal analgesia for controlling acute postoperative pain. Current Opinion in Anesthesiology 2009;22:588–93.

Ilfeld BM, Enneking FK. Continuous peripheral nerve blocks at home: A review. Anesth Analg 2005;100:1822–33.

Joshi GP. Multimodal analgesia techniques for ambulatory surgery. International Anesthesiology Clinics 2005;43:197–204.

Kahn RL, Nelson DA. Regional anesthesia group practice in multihospital private practice settings and in orthopedic specialty hospitals. International Anesthesiology Clinics 2005;43:15–24.

Kehlet H, Liu SS. Continuous local anesthetic wound infusion to improve postoperative outcome-Back to the periphery? Anesthesiology 2007;107:369–71.

Mariano ER, Cheng GS, Choy LP, et al. Electrical stimulation versus ultrasound guidance for popliteal-sciatic perineural catheter insertion. Reg Anesth Pain Med 2009;34:480–85.

McMain L. Principles of acute pain management. Journal of Perioperative Practice 2008;18:472–78.

Sun Y, Gan TJ, Dubose JW, Habib AS. Acupuncture and related techniques for postoperative pain: A systematic review of randomized, controlled trials. Br J Anaesth 2008;101:151–60.

Varrassi G, Donatelli F, Marinangeli F, Paladini A, Rawal N. "Organization of an acute pain service and pain management," in: Raj PP (ed.) *Textbook of Regional Anesthesia*. New York: Churchill Livingstone, 2002. pp. 47–54.

White PF. Multimodal analgesia: Its role in preventing postoperative pain. Current Opinion in Investigational Drugs 2008;9:76–82.

Williams BA, Matusic B, Kentor ML. Regional anesthesia procedures for ambulatory knee surgery: Effects on in-hospital outcomes. International Anesthesiology Clinics 2005;43:153–60.

Williams BA, Motolenich P, Kentor ML. Hospital facilities and resource management: Economic impact of a high-volume regional anesthesia program for outpatients. International Anesthesiology Clinics 2005;43:43–54.

Wu CL. "Efficacy of neuraxial and peripheral nerve blocks in acute pain management," in: Raj PP (ed.) *Textbook of Regional Anesthesia*. New York: Churchill Livingstone, 2002. pp. 873–94.

Index

acetaminophen (Tylenol), 123, 129
acupuncture, 129
adrenaline, 76–77, 108
airway management, 3–4, 33–34, 35, 37, 40; in children, 115; complications of, 52–54; conscious airway placement, 52; guidelines for, 52, 53; for patient with difficult airway, 52–54, 66–67; in pregnancy, 117. *See also* Breathing tube
allergic reaction, 49; to latex, 50; to medications, 9, 24, 49–50, 108
ambulatory surgery, 8, 23, 69; pain control after, 130–31; reasons for prolonged stay after, 13
ambulatory surgical unit, postoperative return to, 12–13
American Association of Nurse Anesthetists, 48
American College of Cardiology, 44
American Heart Association, 44
American Society of Anesthesiologists, 48, 52, 53, 123
American Society of Regional Anesthesia and Pain Medicine, 103, 126
anesthesia: categories of, 1–2, 60; consent for, 9, 10–11, 24, 26, 27, 130; definition of, 2; explaining choices for, 9–11, 21–22, 24; general, 23–40; goal of, 2; history of, 15–22; mortality from, 47, 49, 55; plan for,

45; preoperative evaluation for, 8–9, 23–25, 41–46; preoperative preparation for, 26–27, 32–33; providers of, 1, 3, 4, 5; recovery from, 11–13, 36–37; regional, 60–70; spinal and epidural, 71–82; total intravenous, 34
anesthesia machines, 31
Anesthesia Patient Safety Foundation, 48
anesthesiologist, 1, 3; education and certification of, 5–7; employers of, 8; practice settings for, 7–8
anesthesiology specialty, 5–6, 20
"anesthetic hangover," 13, 39
anesthetics: inhaled, 16–20; local, 20–21; maintenance, 34, 35
anti-anginal agents, 25
antibiotics, allergy to, 49–50
anti-clotting medications, 68, 96, 103
antihistamines, 25
antihypertensives, 25
anti-inflammatory medications, 25, 39, 128, 129, 133
anxiety, preoperative, 26–27
arrhythmias, 43, 110
aspiration, pulmonary, 49, 54, 117
atherosclerosis, 55, 123
awakening from anesthesia, 12, 36
awareness during surgery, 29
axillary nerve block, 116
axons, 85, 126

21, 61; neuraxial, 5, 62, 63, 71–82, 83; peripheral, 5, 61–62, 63, 70, 83–99; for postoperative pain, 10, 14, 39, 40, 62–63, 69–70, 93, 128, 130–31; preoperative, 60–61; with sedation, 66–67; single-shot, 131; transitioning to oral pain medications after, 131. *See also* regional anesthesia

nerve fascicle, anesthetic injection into, 105

nerve injury: during general anesthesia, 105; during regional anesthesia, 104–8

nerve plexuses, 84

neuraxial anesthesia, 5, 62, 63, 71–82, 83; benefits of, 72–73; in children, 115–17; complications of (*see* regional anesthesia complications); in elderly people, 123; obstetric, 9, 71, 78–79, 117–22; for patients who take blood-thinning medications, 103; peripheral nerve blocks and, 83–84, 95–96; procedure for, 73–75; sedation for, 73; surgeries involving, 71, 72; toxicity of local anesthetics for, 110. *See also* epidural anesthesia; spinal anesthesia

neuraxial anesthesia side effects, 80–82; low blood pressure, 80; paresthesias, 80–81; shivering, 81; spinal headache, 81–82

neuropathic pain, 126

neurotransmitters, 127

nitrous oxide, 16, 17–18, 35

nonsteroidal anti-inflammatory drugs, 129

Novocaine (procaine), 2, 61, 75, 108

numbing of body parts. *See* local anesthetics; regional anesthesia

nurse anesthetist, 1, 3, 8

nurses, in PACU, 11–12, 36

obesity, 67

obstetric anesthesia, 2, 71, 117–22; advantages of regional anesthesia,

118, 121–22; for cesarean delivery, 71, 120–21; combined spinal-epidural, 121; dangers of general anesthesia, 117–18; epidural, 9, 78–79, 119–20; fetal deceleration and, 120; history of, 17, 19–20; for labor pain, 119; in pre-eclampsia, 119–20; risks of anesthetic medications, 118; spinal, 120–22; for tubal ligation, 120; uterine blood flow and, 119–20

obstructive sleep apnea (OSA), 67, 122–23

ondansetron (Zofran), 25, 38

operating room, 27–28, 30–33; death in, 49, 57

opioids, 11, 12, 25, 35–36, 39–40; adverse effects of, 39, 67, 123; dementia and, 124; epidural infusion of, 77; for labor and delivery, 119, 121; in patients with obstructive sleep apnea, 122–23; for postoperative pain, 62, 73, 98, 99, 127, 128, 131, 133; preoperative, 27, 129

orthopedic surgery: braces or casts after, 133, 134; continuous regional anesthesia after, 131; epidural anesthesia for, 79, 96–97; immobility after, 127; nerve injury from, 107–8; peripheral nerve blocks for, 94–95, 96–97; reducing blood clots after, 67–68; regional anesthesia for, 67–68, 70

OSA (obstructive sleep apnea), 67, 122–23

outpatient surgery. *See* ambulatory surgery

oxygen/oxygenation, 12, 13, 18, 27, 28, 32, 34, 35, 36, 46, 52, 53, 54, 57, 61, 90, 118, 120

PACU. *See* post-anesthesia care unit

pain, 126; acute vs. chronic, 127; noxious stimuli and wind-up phenomenon, 64–65; perception of, 63–64, 126–27; rating severity of, 127;